Control of Renin Secretion

ADVANCES IN EXPERIMENTAL MEDICINE AND BIOLOGY

Volume 1
THE RETICULOENDOTHELIAL SYSTEM AND ATHEROSCLEROSIS
    Edited by N. R. Di Luzio and R. Paoletti • 1967

Volume 2
PHARMACOLOGY OF HORMONAL POLYPEPTIDES AND PROTEINS
    Edited by N. Back, L. Martini, and R. Paoletti • 1968

Volume 3
GERM-FREE BIOLOGY: Experimental and Clinical Aspects
    Edited by E. A. Mirand and N. Back • 1969

Volume 4
DRUGS AFFECTING LIPID METABOLISM
    Edited by W. L. Holmes, L. A. Carlson, and R. Paoletti • 1969

Volume 5
LYMPHATIC TISSUE AND GERMINAL CENTERS IN IMMUNE RESPONSE
    Edited by L. Fiore-Donati and M. G. Hanna, Jr. • 1969

Volume 6
RED CELL METABOLISM AND FUNCTION
    Edited by George J. Brewer • 1970

Volume 7
SURFACE CHEMISTRY OF BIOLOGICAL SYSTEMS
    Edited by Martin Blank • 1970

Volume 8
BRADYKININ AND RELATED KININS: Cardiovascular, Biochemical, and
Neural Actions
    Edited by F. Sicuteri, M. Rocha e Silva, and N. Back • 1970

Volume 9
SHOCK: Biochemical, Pharmacological, and Clinical Aspects
    Edited by A. Bertelli and N. Back • 1970

Volume 10
THE HUMAN TESTIS
    Edited by E. Rosemberg and C. A. Paulsen • 1970

Volume 11
MUSCLE METABOLISM DURING EXERCISE
    Edited by B. Pernow and B. Saltin • 1971

Volume 12
MORPHOLOGICAL AND FUNCTIONAL ASPECTS OF IMMUNITY
    Edited by K. Lindahl-Kiessling, G. Alm, and M. G. Hanna, Jr. • 1971

Volume 13
CHEMISTRY AND BRAIN DEVELOPMENT
Edited by R. Paoletti and A. N. Davison • 1971

Volume 14
MEMBRANE-BOUND ENZYMES
Edited by G. Porcellati and F. di Jeso • 1971

Volume 15
THE RETICULOENDOTHELIAL SYSTEM AND IMMUNE PHENOMENA
Edited by N. R. Di Luzio and K. Flemming • 1971

Volume 16A
THE ARTERY AND THE PROCESS OF ARTERIOSCLEROSIS: Pathogenesis
Edited by Stewart Wolf • 1971

Volume 16B
THE ARTERY AND THE PROCESS OF ARTERIOSCLEROSIS: Measurement and
Modification
Edited by Stewart Wolf • 1972

Volume 17
CONTROL OF RENIN SECRETION
Edited by Tatiana A. Assaykeen • 1972

Volume 18
THE DYNAMICS OF MERISTEM CELL POPULATIONS
Edited by Morton W. Miller and Charles C. Kuehnert • 1972

Control of Renin Secretion

Proceedings of a Workshop Sponsored by and Held at the
Kroc Foundation, Santa Ynez, California, August 26-29, 1971

Edited by

Tatiana A. Assaykeen

Department of Surgery, Division of Urology
Stanford University School of Medicine
Stanford, California

℗ PLENUM PRESS · NEW YORK-LONDON · 1972

Library of Congress Catalog Card Number 76-185044
ISBN 0-306-39017-5

© 1972   Plenum Press, New York
A Division of Plenum Publishing Corporation
227 West 17th Street, New York, N.Y. 10011

United Kingdom edition published by Plenum Press, London
A Division of Plenum Publishing Company, Ltd.
Davis House (4th Floor), 8 Scrubs Lane, Harlesden, NW10 6SE, London, England

PREFACE

In the summer of 1969, the first Workshop on Control of Renin Secretion was held at Stanford University. At its completion, it was suggested by many of those who attended that a second Workshop be planned in about two years time. Thus the second Workshop on Control of Renin Secretion took place and from this event the chapters in this book had their origin. The setting of this Workshop was the beautiful J & R Double Arch Ranch in Santa Ynez, California which houses the Kroc Foundation. The Foundation, through the kindness of its President, Dr. Robert L. Kroc, provided us with luxurious accommodations, excellent meeting facilities and an atmosphere extremely conducive to the exchange of scientific knowledge, both formally and informally. In addition, the Foundation assisted financially in the travel expenses of three of our foreign guests and in the preparation of the manuscripts for this book. I know I speak for all of us who attended the Workshop in expressing our sincere gratitude to the Foundation and to Dr. and Mrs. Kroc and their staff.

In addition, I personally, as organizer of the meeting and editor, wish to acknowledge the help of many others who made my job much easier. Drs. Davis, Ganong, Luetscher and Tobian kindly took on the jobs of chairing the four sessions and directing the lively discussions which followed each presentation. The lengthy task of retyping the manuscripts for publication was efficiently carried out by Miss P. Schwartz, Miss S. Karsen and Mrs. T. Kovattana who acted not only as typists but as editors as well. And perhaps most importantly, I acknowledge with gratitude the help of Miss B. Leonard and Mrs. J.R. Blair-West in the tedious job of proofreading the final manuscripts. In order to assure publication as rapidly as possible, no galley proofs were sent out and thus the responsibility for proofing the text fell on us. Every effort was made to retype each manuscript accurately and the latter was proofed at least three times. In many cases this process spotted and corrected errors in the original maunscripts as well but we recognize the fact that some errors may have been overlooked inadvertently. We hope that the authors agree with us that the few errors which may

vii

remain are more than balanced by the benefits of rapid publication.

   I think there is no doubt that the Workshop was deemed a
success by those who attended and I hope that the contents of this
book will reflect this to the reader. Since our first meeting two
years ago there have been important advances in the field of renin
control as well as in many areas concerned with the physiological
and pathological role of renin in the body. Many problems still
remain to be solved; hopefully sufficient advances will be made to
warrent a third Workshop in a few years time.

                                        Tatiana A. Assaykeen
October 1971   Stanford, California

CONTENTS

Anatomical Considerations in the Control of Renin Secretion......1
    L. Barajas

Sympathetic Effects on Renin Secretion: Mechanisms and
        Physiological Role....................................17
    W.F. Ganong

The Effects of Cyclic Nucleotides on Plasma Renin Activity and
        Renal Function in Dogs...............................33
    D.J. Allison, H. Tanigawa and T.A. Assaykeen

Effect of Beta-Adrenergic Stimulation on Renin Release.........49
    I.A. Reid, R.W. Schrier and L.E. Earley

Effects of Adrenergic Antagonists in States of Increased Renin
        Secretion..65
    N. Winer, W.G. Walkenhorst, R. Helman and D. Lamy

Renin Secretion, Adrenergic Blockade and Hypertension..........83
    A.M. Michelakis and R.G. McAllister, Jr.

Studies on the Mechanism of Renin Suppression by Alpha-
        Methyldopa...93
    P.J. Privitera and S. Mohammed

Renin Release by Vertebral Artery Embolism....................103
    H. Ueda, Y. Uchida, A. Sakamoto and A. Ebihara

Area Postrema - Angiotensin-Sensitive Site in Brain...........109
    H. Ueda, S. Katayama and R. Kato

The Control of Renin Release in the Non-Filtering Kidney......117
    J.O. Davis, E.H. Blaine, R.T. Witty, J.A. Johnson,
    R.E. Shade and B. Braverman

On the Intrarenal Role of the Renin Angiotensin System.........131
      P. Granger, J.M. Rojo-Ortega, A. Grüner, H. Dahlheim,
      K. Thurau, R. Boucher and J. Genest

Renin Release by Rat Kidney Slices in Vitro....................145
      M.H. Weinberger and D.R. Rosner

Conversion of Angiotensin I to II in Vivo and in Vitro.........151
      S. Oparil and E. Haber

Renal Medullary Mechanisms Relating to Hypertension............159
      L. Tobian, Jr. and S. Azar

The Role of the Renin-Angiotensin System in Control of
      Aldosterone Secretion....................................167
      J.R. Blair-West, J.P. Coghlan, D.A. Denton, J.W. Funder
      and·B.A. Scoggins

Early Morning Variation in Plasma Renin Activity in Normal,
      Recumbent Humans...189
      M.H. Weinberger, D.R. Rosner, D.C. Kem, L. Joyner and
      G. Foust

The Renin-Angiotensin System in Patients Receiving Chronic
      Hemodialysis...193
      M.D. Blaufox, A. Goodman, S. Weseley, H. Schechter and
      E. Weinstein

A Paradoxical Response to Changes in Sodium Intake in Patients
      with Accelerated Hypertension............................209
      P.J. Mulrow, T.A. Kotchen and L.B. Morrow

Low Plasma Renin in Hypertensive Patients: Correlations with
      Aldosterone, Sodium and Potassium Excretion..............217
      J.A. Luetscher and R. Beckerhoff

Mechanisms of Sodium Retention in Congestive Heart Failure.....227
      C.R. Ayers, R.E. Bowden and J.P. Schrank

Hypercalciuria and Increased Plasma Renin Activity.............245
      W.J. Meyer, III, S.A. Middler, C.S. Delea and F.C. Bartter

Acute Circulatory Renal Failure: A Probable Manifestation of
      Excess Renin Release.....................................263
      J.J. Brown, H. Gavras, B. Leckie, A.F. Lever, R. MacAdam,
      J.J. Morton and J.I.S. Robertson

PARTICIPANTS

Donna J. Allison, Department of Physiology, University of
California, San Francisco, California

Tatiana A. Assaykeen, Division of Urology, Stanford University,
Stanford, California

Carlos R. Ayers, Department of Internal Medicine, Division of
Cardiology, University of Virginia, Charlottesville, Virginia

Luciano Barajas, Department of Zoology, University of California,
Los Angeles, California

Reiner Beckerhoff, Department of Medicine, Stanford University,
Stanford, California

John R. Blair-West, Howard Florey Institute of Experimental
Physiology and Medicine, University of Melbourne, Parkville,
Australia

M. Donald Blaufox, Departments of Medicine and Radiology, Albert
Einstein College of Medicine, Bronx, New York

James O. Davis, Department of Physiology, University of Missouri,
Columbia, Missouri

Derek A. Denton, Howard Florey Institute of Experimental Physiology
and Medicine, University of Melbourne, Parkville, Australia

William F. Ganong, Department of Physiology, University of
California, San Francisco, California

Pierre Granger, Clinical Research Institute of Montreal, Montreal,
Quebec, Canada

Edgar Haber, Cardiac Unit, Medical Services, Massachusetts General
Hospital and the Department of Medicine, Harvard Medical School,
Boston, Massachusetts

John A. Luetscher, Department of Medicine, Stanford University, Stanford, California

Walter J. Meyer, III, Endocrinology Branch, National Heart and Lung Institute, Bethesda, Maryland

Andrew M. Michelakis, Departments of Medicine and Pharmacology, Vanderbilt University School of Medicine, Nashville, Tennessee

Patrick J. Mulrow, Department of Internal Medicine, Yale University School of Medicine, New Haven, Connecticut

Philip J. Privitera, Division of Clinical Pharmacology, Departments of Medicine and Pharmacology, University of Cincinnati College of Medicine, Cincinnati, Ohio

Ian A. Reid, Department of Physiology, University of California, San Francisco, California

J. Ian S. Robertson, Medical Research Council, Blood Pressure Unit, Western Infirmary, Glasgow, Scotland

Morris Schambelan, Clinical Study Center, San Francisco General Hospital, San Francisco, California

Hiromi Tanigawa, Division of Urology, Stanford University, Stanford, California

Louis Tobian, Jr., Department of Medicine, University of Minnesota, Minneapolis, Minnesota

Hideo Ueda, Second Department of Internal Medicine, University of Tokyo, Tokyo, Japan

Myron H. Weinberger, Renal Hypertension Laboratory, Department of Medicine, Indiana University School of Medicine, Indianapolis, Indiana

Edward Weinstein, Departments of Medicine and Radiology, Albert Einstein College of Medicine, Bronx, New York

Nathaniel Winer, Department of Medicine, Menorah Medical Center, Kansas City, Missouri

ANATOMICAL CONSIDERATIONS IN THE CONTROL OF RENIN SECRETION

L. Barajas

Department of Zoology, University of California

Los Angeles, California

At the hilus of the renal glomerulus a portion of the distal tubule changes its morphologic characteristics and establishes a special relationship with the vascular pole. This observation dates back to Golgi's time (14) and has been repeatedly confirmed by many histologists beginning with the work of Peter (35). The precise morphologic description of this relationship, however, remained vague because of two technically limiting factors: 1) the resolution of the light microscope which is not sufficient to clearly outline the structures involved; and 2) sectioning methods capable of producing only relatively thick sections and soft embedding media which made the sections susceptible to compression, leading to artefactual contact between unrelated structures.

Another important observation made by early workers was the presence of large collections of cytoplasmic granules in the cells of the media of the afferent arteriole as it approached the glomerulus. These granules were first observed in the afferent arteriole of the mouse by Ruyter in 1925 (38) and soon after that were described in man by Oberling (30). They have been demonstrated in many other species by a variety of staining methods (32,33). One of the best of the juxtaglomerular granule stains was developed by the Hartrofts as a modification of the Bowie method (18). Their technique is very reproducible and has been extremely useful in quantitative determinations of degrees of granularity.

In the late thirties Goormaghtigh (15,16) suggested that the granule-containing cells of the arteriole and the distal tubule might work as a functional unit and proposed the concept of the juxtaglomerular apparatus (although he applied the term exclusively to the vascular component). His theory included two assumptions: 1) that the granular cells of the arteriolar wall contained renin; and 2) that the distal tubular segment associated with them acted as a

1

sensitive plaque which controlled the function of the adjacent granular cells. The relationship between the distal tubule and the granular cells thus became fundamental to the whole concept of the JG
apparatus. Light microscopists imvestigated this problem, but because of the above mentioned technical limitations their results were
inconclusive. All of them reported contact between the afferent arteriole (and granular cells) and a group of cells located between the
arterioles, the so-called juxtaglomerular body (Polkissen, laci) (56,
31). Some authors (11,24,26,27) described occasional contact involving the efferent arteriole. De Castro and de la Pena (11), the only
ones to illustrate such a contact, called it an "atypical juxtaglomerular apparatus."

     In summary it can be said that in the late 50's the JG apparatus
was commonly (and as we now know, erroneously) understood to be formed essentially by contact between the afferent arteriole and the
attached distal tubule.

The Role of Electron Microscopy

     Tissue section electron microscopy is ideally suited to the
study of the JG apparatus from two standpoints: 1) the resolution
required to investigate the structures (basement membranes and cell
processes) involved in the contact is easily obtained; and 2) the
hard plastics in which the tissue is embedded for electron microscopy greatly decreases compression and with it the possibility of
false contact. Initially the largest obstacle to be overcome is the
finding of the JG apparatus which is like finding the proverbial
needle in a haystack.

     In 1960, Oberling and Hatt (31) were the first to report an
electron microscopic study of the JG apparatus. In their excellent
paper they report extensive and intimate contact of the JG body
(they called it laci or lacework because it is formed by the inter-
mingling of cellular processes), with the distal tubule. They also
described membrane-bound granules in the arteriolar wall and noted
the similarity of these granules to secretory granules found elsewhere. Their findings were confirmed by Hartroft and Newmark (19),
Latta and Maunsbach (22), and others. Since then electron microscopy
has continued to provide strong morphological evidence of the endocrine nature of the granular cells. The most compelling examples
come from the hypergranulated ischemic kidneys of patients with renovascular hypertension (7) (Figures 1 and 2). In some instances a
newly recognized granular form, a protogranule, appears to occupy
large portions of the cytoplasm. These protogranules have a clear
origin from the Golgi region, exhibit crystalline substructure, are
of rhomboidal shape and are separated by a halo from the surrounding
membrane (2,6,7). Their similarity to beta cell granules of the
pancreatic islets is striking (21). They seem to be the precursors

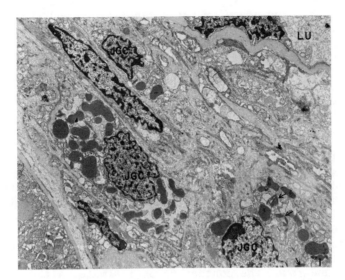

Figure 1. A portion of the hyper-granulated afferent arteriole of
the juxtaglomerular apparatus of an "ischemic" kidney
of a patient with renovascular hypertension. The lumen
of the arteriole appears in the upper right (LU) and
several granular cells (JGC) are observed in the photograph. In the lower right part of the picture several
protogranules (→) can be seen. (16,000 X).(Reprinted
with permission from Hosp. Prac. 4:53, 1969)

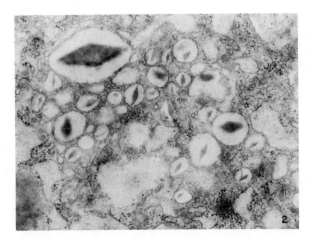

Figure 2. A photograph at higher magnification of the cytoplasm
of a granular cell from the same patient. A concentration of crystal-shaped protogranules surrounded by a
clear halo can be seen. The resemblance to beta cell
granules of the pancreas is striking. (60,000 X).

of the large irregular "typical" JG granules. An increasing body
of evidence that the granular cells manufacture and store renin
has accumulated over the last two decades (10,13,20,34).

My own contribution started in the laboratory of Harrison Latta
where I began looking at the JG apparatus with the light microscope
using the newly developed technique of toluidine blue staining of
plastic-embedded tissue (8). As I looked for the arterioles at the
hilus of the glomerulus, each time I found an arteriole it was
either full of granular cells or in contact with the distal tubule.
Since both these criteria were supposed to define the afferent
arteriole I began to wonder where the efferent arteriole was. To
answer this question serial sections approximately 1µ thick of the
Epon-embedded blocks were cut and a free-hand model constructed (5).
It showed an area of extensive contact between the distal tubule
and the efferent arteriole and very little, if any, with the afferent arteriole, where most of the granules were. This finding raised
the question of the validity of Goormaghtigh's macula densa hypothesis. We looked at thin sections of the series with the electron
microscope and found the contact to be intimate, although always
separated by basement membrane material and by a distance of
between 1000-2000 Å. The limitations of the light microscope,
however, did not allow us to see exactly what was between the arterioles and the distal tubule along most of the area of contact. The
very irregular shape of the cells and their long processes made it
risky to draw conclusions from the light microscopic analysis regarding the extent of contact, even with electron microscopic observations sandwiched among the semifine serial sections. I therefore
reluctantly resorted to serial section electron microscopy.

                The Electron Microscopy Serial Section Technique

This rather laborious technique has been most extensively used,
and in large part developed, in Dr. F.S. Sjostrand's laboratory,
so I moved there to learn it (41).

Preparatory methods and methods of three-dimensional recon-
struction have been discussed in more detail elsewhere (3); briefly,
I used kidneys fixed either by perfusion with 1% glutaraldehyde in
phosphate buffer followed by immersion in 1% phosphate-buffered
osmium tetroxide, or by dripping on the kidney in situ and later
immersion of fixed pieces in 1% phosphate-buffered osmium tetroxide.
The tissue was embedded in Vestopal, the only embedding medium we
found capable of giving the long series of thin serial sections
required.

A critical part of the preparatory technique was the preliminary sectioning required to locate a whole JG apparatus. An MT-1
ultramicrotome was used for most of this semithin sectioning.

Initially the largest block face possible, including the kidney capsule for orientation, was cut. The semithin sections were stained with toluidine blue. After some time I could anticipate the appearance of a JG apparatus in the light microscopic serial sections and start the ribbons of thin sections before any contact between the arterioles and the distal tubule had started. The sections were mounted on Formvar-coated single-hole copper grids. Series of 500 sections were required.

Since the region of the JG apparatus is too large to be contained in one electron micrograph, montages of each section had to be made (Figure 3a). Hundreds of these large montages were required, but at last we could see the whole unit at the electron microscope level. These hundreds of montages created a serious space problem. A storage method we found very helpful was the use of commercial clothes racks with wheels. This enabled us to borrow space and realistically promise to clear it on 24 hours notice.

A Definition of the Juxtaglomerular Apparatus

Before we could begin an analysis of the JG apparatus it was necessary to introduce a definition of its boundaries. The JG apparatus was considered to have two components, the vascular and tubular. The vascular component included: 1) those portions of the afferent and efferent arterioles from the point where the granular cells away from the glomerulus first make their appearance to the glomerular hilus; and 2) the extraglomerular mesangial and arteriolar areas in contact with the distal tubule. The tubular component was that part of the distal tubule in contact with the vascular components.

Three-Dimensional Analysis

In order to measure the surfaces of contact between the distal tubule and the vascular components a fairly accurate estimate of the thickness of the sections was required. Fortunately, the kidney has large numbers of spherical bodies of a lysosomal nature throughout the proximal convoluted tubule. By measuring their diameter and counting the number of sections required to go through an entire body the average section thickness was found to be 850 ± 100 Å.

Once the section thickness was known the surface of contact could be easily calculated. The line of contact was measured in the electron micrographs by rolling a map measurer over it; the surface of contact was then obtained by multiplying this one-dimensional measurement by the section thickness.

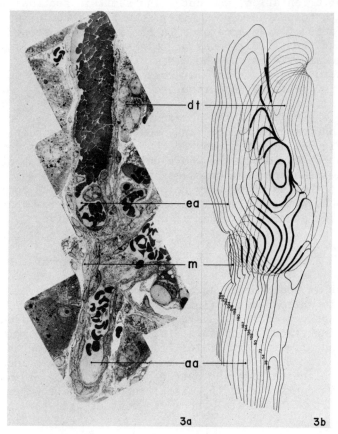

Figure 3.   (a) A montage of electron micrographs from JG 2. The
             distal tubule appears in contact with the efferent
             arteriole in the upper part of the picture. The
             afferent arteriole appears at the lower part of the
             picture, entering into the glomerulus in the center of
             the photograph. The mesangial region separates the
             arterioles. Granular cells are present in both
             arterioles. (1,000 X). (b) Three-dimensional recon-
             struction of the JG 2 section series. It was con-
             structed by superimposing schematic drawings of every
             18th section. The areas in which contact occurs are
             represented by thick lines; the different components of
             the juxtaglomerular apparatus are outlined in thin
             lines. In the lower portion of the illustration the
             lines are numbered according to their corresponding
             sections. Distal tubule (dt), mesangial region (m),
             afferent arteriole (aa), and efferent arteriole (ea).
             (1,000 X) (Reprinted with permission from Sci.172:
             485, 1971)

TABLE I*

Surface of Contact Between the Vascular and Tubular
Components of the Juxtaglomerular Apparatus

Contact of the distal tubule with:

	Efferent Art.	Afferent Art.	Mesangial	Total
JG-1	601 μ^2	43 μ^2	267 μ^2	911 μ^2
JG-2	549 μ^2	--	633 μ^2	1182 μ^2
JG-3	374 μ^2	--	547 μ^2	921 μ^2
JG-4	710 μ^2	68 μ^2	912 μ^2	1690 μ^2

---

* Reprinted with permission from J. Ultrastr. Res. 33:116, 1970.

The surfaces of contact of four JG apparatuses were measured
(Table I). These measurements confirmed our light microscopic
observations of prolonged contact between the efferent arteriole
and the distal tubule. The distance between the two components at
the site of contact was 1000-2000 Å. Another central feature which
emerged from this study was an appreciation of the extent and
nature of the contact between the distal tubule and the extraglomerular mesangium (polkissen of Zimmerman, laci of Oberling,
juxtaglomerular body of McManus). It was in this area that cellular
cytoplasmic projections of one component into the other with fusion
and continuity of their basement membranes were seen. This was in
contrast to the arteriolartubular contact which consisted mainly of
simple apposition of the basement membranes. The occurrence of two
distinct types of contact seemed to indicate the possibility that
this arrangement had important physiological significance; a point
which I will enlarge upon later.

Construction of a Three-Dimensional Model

Two factors had to be considered in the planning of the model:
one, of course, was accuracy and the other was readability. A
physical model was first considered and rejected. Solid structures,
no matter how transparent, would invariably obstruct important views

when mounted together. Instead we began by building a graphic model
to illustrate the relationship between the tubular and vascular
components. The gross outlines of the montages were traced on to
transparent plastic Mylar sheets. The lines of contact were thick-
ened for emphasis. These two-dimensional representations of each
section were then superimposed and offset a consistent amount to
give a three-dimensional representation (Figure 3b). By this method
we could draw models of the tubular and vascular components separately, mounted together, or of the area of contact alone. More
details of the methods involved and illustrations of the models are
given elsewhere (3).

Juxtaglomerular Cell Distribution by Granularity and Distal Tubular Contact

When the study of the areas of contact was completed we pro-
ceeded to the analysis of the tubular and vascular cells themselves
and their relation to each other (4).

Each of the cells of the vascular component was characterized
as to position (afferent arteriole, mesangium, efferent arteriole)
and granularity, and its nucleus located and numbered on the montages. The cells were then traced through the series of montages
to establish whether or not they contacted the macula densa. This
data for four JG apparatuses is shown in Table II. A new and interesting finding was that the majority of the granular cells are not
in contact with the distal tubule. In one JG apparatus there was
no contact at all between the granular cells and the distal tubule.

An Interpretation (3,4)

As was stated above, at the extraglomerular mesangial region
there are projections from the bases of the cells of the distal
tubule penetrating into the vascular component with fusion and
network formation of the basement membranes. I have considered
this type of contact to be permanent and to represent the site at
which the distal tubule is anchored to the vascular component. The
type of contact involving a simple adjacency of basement membranes
I have interpreted to be reversible. Although the variations in
contact reported here may be due to the different responses of
individual nephrons to the preparatory techniques, the fact that
most of the granular cells are located where contact, if any, would
be reversible, indicates that variations in contact may occur under
normal physiological conditions.

Current theories have implicated either changes in sodium concentration at the distal tubule (macula densa theory) (28,39,44,45,
50,51,53,55) or changes in the volume and stretch of the afferent

TABLE II *

Juxtaglomerular Cell Distribution by Granularity
and Distal Tubular Contact

JG Apparatus Cell Location	Agranular Cell Count Contact	Agranular Cell Count No Contact	Granular Cell Count Contact	Granular Cell Count No Contact	TOTAL
JG - 1					
mesangial	6	8	0	3	17
efferent arteriole	5	13	7	6	31
afferent arteriole	0	5	1	10	16
TOTAL	11	26	8	19	64
JG - 2					
mesangial	15	17	1	1	34
efferent arteriole	2	25	2	9	38
afferent arteriole	0	9	0	13	22
TOTAL	17	51	3	23	94
JG - 3					
mesangial	15	19	0	3	37
efferent arteriole	2	10	0	0	12
afferent arteriole	0	4	0	11	15
TOTAL	17	33	0	14	64
JG - 4					
mesangial	17	17	0	5	39
efferent arteriole	8	10	0	1	19
afferent arteriole	0	21	1	14	36
TOTAL	25	48	1	20	94

* Reprinted with permission from Sci. 172:485, 1971 (slightly
  modified).

arteriole (stretch receptor theory) (42,43,46,47) as the factors
which control renin secretion. A model based on the anatomical
findings presented here and previously,in which variations in contact between the elements of the JG apparatus are responsible for
the control of renin secretion,may unify the supporting evidence
for both theories.

With regard to the macula densa theory, many physiologists
interpret their data as indicating that lowered sodium transport
through the distal tubule increases renin secretion. A smaller
sodium load in the distal tubule would probably be accompanied by
a decrease in its volume and therefore decreased contact with granular cells. This mechanism also fits the stretch receptor theory
which is based on the fact that lowering the blood volume passing
through the arterioles increases renin secretion and vice versa
(Figure 4a and 4b). Provisionally we can propose that less contact
leads to an increase while more contact decreases renin secretion.
The basic mechanisms are still unknown, however it is probable that
whatever chemical influence the distal tubule exerts on the granular
cells will be altered by changes in contact.

In addition, it should be noted that there are granular cells
so far removed from the distal tubule that any contact between them
seems unlikely. These granular cells are occasionally seen to be
in contact with the proximal tubule and reversible contact between
some of these cells and the proximal tubule may be possible. To
what extent the proximal tubule participates in the control of renin
secretion is unknown but, on strictly anatomical grounds, it is
possible that physiological changes in the proximal tubule could
modify renin secretion.

Electron Microscopy and the Question of the Innervation
of the JG Apparatus

In our previous scheme we have simplified things by ignoring
the role of the nerves in the function of the JG apparatus. We
can denervate the kidney easily enough in our drawings, but it is
probably more difficult to do so in reality.

A rich innervation of the glomerular arterioles and a more
debatable innervation of the tubular system was described by the
light microscopists using a large variety of stains. (For an
excellent summary of the situation up to 1952 regarding the
existence and distribution of nerves and nerve endings by light
microscopy, see the review by DeMuylder (12).) With the advent of
electron microscopy a number of questions posed by the light microscopists were easily answered in the negative: 1) are there myelin-
ated nerves in the hilus of the glomerulus? and 2) do nerves enter
the glomerular tuft?

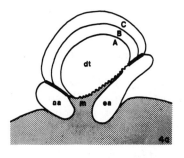

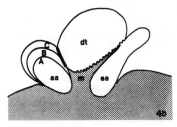

Figure 4.   A simplified schematic representation of the proposed
            functional model of the juxtaglomerular apparatus.
            The contact between the distal tubule (dt) and the
            mesangial region (m) and the hilar efferent arteriole
            (ea) which is interpreted as permanent is represented
            by wavy lines, whereas the reversible type of contact
            is represented by heavy lines. (4a) As the distal
            tubule expands (lines B and C) the area of "reversible"
            contact with the vascular components increases, and
            (4b) representation of the changes in contact between
            the distal tubule and the afferent arterioles result-
            ing from changes in the volume of the afferent arteri-
            ole. (Reprinted with permission from Sci. 172:485,1971)

    The situation with regard to the innervation of the JG apparatus
was complicated rather than clarified when the first electron microscopic papers reported the total absence of nerves. At this time
nerves were also difficult to find in other vessels (36). Where
then was the rich innervation reported by the light microscopists?

    When I began my own electron microscopic study of the JG
innervation in the rat I initially found only occasional nerve-like
structures. Later, in the examination of renal biopsies from
patients with renovascular hypertension, I found a large number of
unquestionable nerve fibers. The preservation of the tissue was
not good enough for critical electron microscopic studies, so a
study of the JG apparatus of the monkey and rat was undertaken (1).
The extensive innervation reported by the light microscopists

became very obvious. All the nerves seen were unmyelinated and no
nerves were seen penetrating into the glomerulus. Nerve endings
were seen reaching granular cells as well as non-granular cells,
and the rich innervation of the vascular component was established.

Many of the nerve endings had the morphologic characteristics
attributed to the adrenergic type. These findings have been confirmed by Simpson and Devine (40) and more recently by others (23,
37). The histochemical fluorescence method for biogenic monoamines
was first applied to the kidney by Nilsson who showed a good adrenergic innervation of the afferent arteriole in the rat (29). These
observations were confirmed and extended by McKenna and Angelakos
(25). More recently Wagermark et al.(54) have elegantly demonstrated sympathetic nerve endings on the granular cells by combining
the histochemical fluorescence method with Bowie staining of the
same sections.

Innervation of the macula densa was reported by Hartroft (17).
I have also seen nerves in the macula densa (Figure 5). Their
contact is very similar to that reported for the arterioles, with
fusion of the two basement membranes and distances of about 2000Å
between the plasma membrane of the tubular cell and that of the
nerve ending.

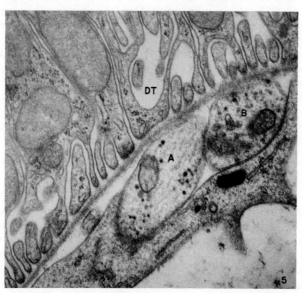

Figure 5.   Two nerve endings (A and B) contacting the distal
            tubule at the hilus of the glomerulus. The dense-
            cored vesicles are of the type associated with
            adrenergic nerves. (51,000 X).

Anatomical proof of the existence of a rich innervation of the area has stimulated interest in the physiological role of nerves in the control of renin secretion (9,48,49,52). Since nerve endings have been found contacting granular cells as well as the smooth muscle cells of the arterioles, one can visualize two possible neural effects on the secretion of renin: 1) direct stimulation of the granular cells, and 2) producing contraction of the smooth muscle cells which would reduce the contact between the macula densa and the arterioles thereby altering secretion by the previously outlined contact theory.

ACKNOWLEDGEMENTS

I am very grateful to my student Jacqueline Müller for her assistance in the preparation of this manuscript. The work reported was supported by U.S. Public Health Research Grant R01 HE 11114 from the National Heart Institute.

REFERENCES

1. Barajas, L. The innervation of the juxtaglomerular apparatus. An electron microscopic study of the innervation of the glomerular arterioles. Lab. Invest. 13: 916-929, 1964.
2. Barajas, L., The development and ultrastructure of the juxtaglomerular cell granule. J. Ultrastruct. Res. 15: 400-413, 1966.
3. Barajas, L., The ultrastructure of the juxtaglomerular apparatus as disclosed by three-dimensional reconstructions from serial sections. The anatomical relationship between the tubular and vascular components. J. Ultrastruct. Res. 33: 116-147, 1970.
4. Barajas, L., Renin secretion: An anatomical basis for tubular control. Science 172: 485, 1971.
5. Barajas, L. and H. Latta, A three-dimensional study of the juxtaglomerular apparatus in the rat. Light and electron microscopic observations. Lab. Invest. 12: 257-269, 1963.
6. Barajas, L. and H. Latta, The development of the juxtaglomerular cell granule. Anat. Rec. 151: 321, 1965.
7. Barajas, L., R.J. Sampson and H. Latta, The juxtaglomerular apparatus of patients with renovascular hypertension: light and electron microscopic study. Fed. Proc. 24: 435, 1965.
8. Bencosme, S.A., R.S. Stone, H. Latta and S.C. Madden, A rapid method for localization of tissue structures or lesions for electron microscopy. J. Biophys. & Biochem. Cytol. 5: 508-510, 1959.
9. Birbari, A., Effect of sympathetic nervous system on renin release. Am. J. Physiol. 220: 16, 1971.
10. Cook, W.F., The detection of renin in juxtaglomerular cells. J. Physiol. (London) 194: 73-4p, 1968.

11. De Castro, F. and A. de la Pena, Sobre la estructura y significacion de la macula densa y organo yuxtaglomerular de rinon humano. Rev. Clin. Esp. 46: 350-359, 1952.

12. De Muylder, C.G., The "Neurility" of the Kidney. A monograph on nerve supply to the kidney. (Charles C. Thomas, Springfield, Ill., 1952).

13. Edelman, R. and P.M. Hartroft, Localization of renin in juxtaglomerular cells of rabbit and dog through the use of fluorescent antibody technique. Circ. Res. 9: 1069-1077, 1961.

14. Golgi, C., Annotazioni intorno all'istologia dei reni dell'uomo e di altri mammiferi e sulla istogenesi dei calalicoli uriniferi. Atti R Acad. dei Lincei, Sez IV, Rendiconti 5: 334, 1889.

15. Goormaghtigh, N., Existence of an endocrine gland in the media of the renal arterioles. Proc. Soc. Exp. Biol. Med. 42: 688-689, 1939.

16. Goormaghtigh. N., La fonction endocrine des arterioles renales: son role dans la pathogenie de l'hypertension arterielle. Rev. Belge Sci. Med. 16: 65, 1945.

17. Hartroft, P.M., Electron microscopy of nerve endings associated with juxtaglomerular cells and macula densa. Lab. Invest. 15: 1127, 1966.

18. Hartroft, P.M. and W.S. Hartroft, Studies on renal juxtaglomerular cells: I. Variations produced by sodium chloride and desoxycortisone acetate. J. Exp. Med. 97: 415, 1953.

19. Hartroft, P.M. and L.N. Newmark, Electron microscopy of renal juxtaglomerular cells. Anat. Rec. 139: 185, 1961.

20. Hartroft, P.M., L.E. Sutherland and W.S. Hartroft, Juxtaglomerular cells as the source of renin: Further studies with the fluorescent antibody technique and the effect of passive transfer of antirenin. Can. Med. Assoc. J. 90: 163, 1964.

21. Herman, L., T. Sato and P. Fitzgerald. In: Electron Microscopic Anatomy, ed. by S. Kurtz. (Academic Press, New York, 1964), p. 59.

22. Latta, H. and A.B. Maunsbach, The juxtaglomerular apparatus as studied electron microscopically. J. Ultrastr. Res. 6: 547-561, 1962.

23. Learanth, C., G. Unguary and T. Donath, The innervation of the juxtaglomerular apparatus. Acta Morph. Acad. Sci. Hung. 17: 131-141, 1969.

24. Martuzzi, M., La Macula Densa Nella Patologia Renale, ed. by Capelli, (Arti Grafiche, Rocca San Cascino, 1955).

25. McKenna, O.C. and E.T. Angelakos, Adrenergic innervation of the canine kidney. Circ. Res. 22: 345-354, 1968.

26. Mc Manus, J.F.A., Juxtaglomerular complex. Lancet 2: 394, 1942.

27. Mc Manus, J.F.A., Apparent reversal of position of the Golgi element in the renal tubule. Nature (London) 152: 417, 1943.

28. Meyer, P., J. Menard, N. Papanicolaou, J-M. Alexandre, C. Devaux and P. Milliez, Mechanism of renin release following furosemide diuresis in rabbit. Am. J. Physiol. 215: 908-915, 1968.

29. Nilsson, O., Adrenergic innervation of the kidney. Lab. Invest. 14: 1392, 1965.
30. Oberling, C., L'existence d'une housse neuromusculaire au niveau des artères glomérulaires de l'homme. C.R. Acad. Sci., Paris 184: 1200-02, 1927.
31. Oberling, C. and P.Y. Hatt, Etude de l'appareil juxtaglomerulaire du rat au microscope electronique. Ann. Anat. Path. (Paris) 5: 441-474, 1960.
32. Okkels, H.M., Sur l'existence d'une spécialisation morphologique au diveau du pole vasculaire du glomérule renale chez la granouille. C.R. Acad. Sci., Paris 188: 193, 1929.
33. Okkels, H.M. and T. Peterfi, Beobachtungen über die Glomerulus= gefässe der Froschniere. Z. Zellforsch. 9: 327-331, 1929.
34. Page, I.H. and J.W. Mc Cubbin, Renal Hypertension. (Year Book Medical Publishers, Inc., Chicago, Ill., 1968)
35. Peter, K., Die Nierenkanalchen des Menschen und einiger Sauge= tiere. Anat. Anz. 30: 114-124, 1907.
36. Rhodin, J.A.G., Fine structure of vascular walls in mammals with special reference to smooth muscle component. Physiol. Rev. 42 (Suppl. 5): 48, 1962.
37. Rojo-Ortega, J.M., P.Y. Hatt and J. Genest, Apropos of the innervation of the juxtaglomerular cells. Electron microscope study in different experimental conditions in rats. Path. Biol. 16: 497-504, 1968.
38. Ruyter, J.H., Über einer merkwürdigen Abschnitt der Vasa Afferentia in der Mänsniere. Z. Zellforsch. 2: 242, 1925.
39. Schnermann, J., Microperfusion study of single short loops of Henle in rat kidney. Pflugers Archiv. 300: 255-282, 1968.
40. Simpson, F.O. and C.E. Devine, The fine structure of autonomic neuromuscular contacts in arterioles of sheep renal cortex. J. Anat. 100: 127-137, 1966.
41. Sjostrand, F.S., Electron Microscopy of Cells and Tissues. (Academic Press, New York, 1967).pp. 370-381, 287-294.
42. Skinner, S.L., J.L. McCubbin and I.H. Page, Angiotensin in blood and lymph following reduction in renal arterial perfusion pressure in dogs. Circ. Res. 13: 336, 1963a.
43. Skinner, S.L., J.L. McCubbin and I.H. Page, Renal baroreceptor control of renin secretion. Science 141: 184, 1963b.
44. Thurau, K., Influence of sodium concentration at macula densa cells on tubular sodium load. Ann. N.Y. Acad. Sci. 139: 388-399, 1966.
45. Thurau, K., J. Schnermann, W. Nagel, M. Horster and M. Wahl, Composition of tubular fluid in the macula densa segment as a factor regulating the function of the juxtaglomerular apparatus. Circ. Res. Suppl. II, 20: 11-79, 1967.
46. Tobian, L., Physiology of the juxtaglomerular cells. Ann. Int. Med. 52: 395-410, 1960.
47. Tobian, L., J. Janecek and A. Tomboulian, Correlation between granulation of juxtaglomerular cells and extractable renin in rats with experimental hypertension. Proc. Soc. Expt. Biol. Med. 100: 94, 1959.

48. Vander, A.J., Effect of catecholamines and renal nerves on renin secretion in anesthetized dogs. Am. J. Physiol. 209: 659-662, 1965.
49. Vander, A.J., Nature of the stimulus for renin secretion in anesthetized dogs. Hypertension (Am. Heart Assoc. Monograph) 13: 126-130, 1965.
50. Vander, A.J., Control of renin release. Physiol. Rev. 47:359-382, 1967.
51. Vander, A.J. and J. Carlson, Mechanism of the effects of furosemide on renin secretion in anesthetized dogs. Circ. Res. 25: 145, 1969.
52. Vander, A.J. and J.R. Luciano, Neural and humoral control of renin release in salt depletion. Hypertension (Am. Heart Assoc. Monograph) 15: 69, 1967.
53. Vander, A.J. and R. Miller, Control of renin secretion in the anesthetized dog. Am. J. Physiol. 207: 537, 1964.
54. Wagermark, J., U. Ungerstedt and A. Ljunqvist, Sympathetic innervation of the juxtaglomerular cells of the kidney. Circ. Res. 22: 149-153, 1968.
55. White, F.N., Control of renin secretion in the dog. Circ. Res. 32: 11-19, 1965.
56. Zimmermann, K.W., Über der Bau des Glomerulus der Saugerniere. Z. Mikr. Anat. Forsch. 32: 176-278, 1933.

SYMPATHETIC EFFECTS ON RENIN SECRETION: MECHANISM

AND PHYSIOLOGICAL ROLE

W. F. Ganong

Department of Physiology, University of California

San Francisco, California

Considerable evidence indicates that renin secretion is regulated in part via the sympathetic nervous system. The sympathetic
effects appear to be mediated by way of β-adrenergic receptors
that are probably located in the kidneys. Indeed, there is reason to believe that circulating catecholamines and norepinephrine
liberated at adrenergic nerve terminals near the juxtaglomerular
cells act directly on these secretory cells to stimulate renin
secretion. In the present paper, I would like to review the
evidence for these statements and analyze the physiological role
of the sympathetic nervous system in the regulation of renin
secretion.

It was first observed some years ago by Vander and by others
that infusion of catecholamines and stimulation of the renal nerves
increased renin secretion (for references see Assaykeen and
Ganong, 1971). We subsequently found that insulin-induced hypoglycemia stimulated renin secretion, and that although the response was unaffected by renal denervation, it was markedly reduced by adrenal denervation (Otsuka et al., 1970). This suggested that the increase was secondary to increased adrenal medullary secretion. The response to hypoglycemia was potentiated by
the α-adrenergic blocking drug, phenoxybenzamine, while it was
essentially abolished by the β-adrenergic blocking drug, propranolol (Assaykeen et al., 1970). Additional evidence that sympathetic
stimulation can increase renin secretion was provided by the observation that stimulation of the pressor region of the medulla
oblongata produces an increase in renin secretion (Passo et al.,
1971a). Such stimulation produces a marked rise in blood pressure
and a marked fall in glomerular filtration rate (Wise and Ganong,

1960). The increase in renin secretion and the decrease in glomerular filtration rate are both blocked by renal denervation. However, the renin response is unaffected by phenoxybenzamine which is reported to block sympathetic effects on the renal vasculature (Gump et al., 1968), and is markedly reduced or abolished by propranolol (Passo et al., 1971b). The renin-stimulating effect of epinephrine is also potentiated by phenoxybenzamine and blocked by propranolol (Assaykeen et al., 1970). In our experiments, epinephrine infusions at a rate of 0.27 and 0.6 μg/kg/min increased plasma renin activity. Infusion of norepinephrine at a rate of 0.6 μg/kg/min had no effect on plasma renin activity (Otsuka et al., 1970). Others have reported increased renin secretion when norepinephrine was infused in bigger doses, and it is possible that the rise in renin secretion produced by this catecholamine is in part secondary to renal vasoconstriction with a decline in glomerular filtration rate and decreased sodium excretion (Ueda et al., 1971). A number of investigators have reported that isoproterenol, a catecholamine with strong β agonist activity, increases renin secretion (for references see Assaykeen and Ganong, 1971). Allison et al. (1970) have shown that this increase is apparently potentiated by α-adrenergic blockade and that it is abolished by β-adrenergic blockade. The effects of β-adrenergic stimulation are believed to be mediated by cyclic AMP (Robison and Sutherland, 1970), and cyclic AMP and dibutyrl cyclic AMP have been reported to stimulate renin secretion when injected into the renal artery (Winer et al., 1969; Allison and Assaykeen, unpublished observations). Finally, theophylline increases renin secretion and this increase is unaffected by α- or β-adrenergic blockade (Reid and Ganong, 1971). This response would be expected if renin secretion was increased by β-adrenergic stimulation, since the methyl xanthine theophylline increases intracellular cyclic AMP (Robison and Sutherland, 1970).

All these data are consistent with the hypothesis that the sympathetic nervous system increases renin secretion by way of β-adrenergic receptors. The data are summarized in Table I.

Where are the β-adrenergic receptors that affect renin secretion located and how do they trigger renin release? The site of the receptors is a matter of some recent debate, but considerable evidence indicates that they are in the kidney. Evidence supporting this conclusion is the observation by Ayers et al. (1969) that isoproterenol has a greater renin-stimulating effect when it is injected into a renal artery than when it is injected intravenously.

Another piece of evidence in favor of the intrarenal location of the receptors is the finding that the increase in renin secretion produced by stimulation of the renal nerves is blocked by propranolol. J. Loeffler, J.R. Stockigt and I found that two

TABLE I

Evidence that Sympathetic Stimulation Increases Renin

Secretion via a β-Receptor Mechanism

1. The increase in renin secretion produced by hypo-
    glycemia is potentiated by phenoxybenzamine and
    inhibited by propranolol.

2. The increase in renin secretion produced by stimu-
    lation of the brain stem is unaffected by phenoxy-
    benzamine and markedly reduced by propranolol.

3. The increase in renin secretion produced by in-
    fusing epinephrine or isoproterenol is potentiated
    by phenoxybenzamine and abolished by propranolol.

4. The renin-stimulating activity of epinephrine
    and isoproterenol is greater than that of norepi-
    nephrine.

5. Dibutyrl cyclic AMP stimulates renin secretion.

6. Theophylline produces an increase in renin se-
    cretion that is unaffected by phenoxybenzamine or
    propranolol.

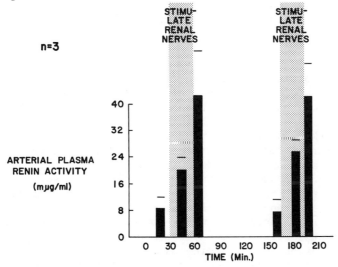

Figure 1.   Effect of renal nerve stimulation on plasma renin
            activity in dogs. Plasma renin activity measured by
            bioassay.

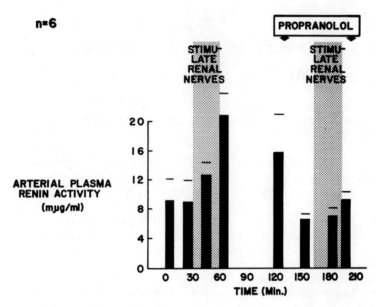

Figure 2.   Effect of propranolol on the renin response to renal
            nerve stimulation in dogs.   Renin measured by bioassay.
            From Assaykeen and Ganong, 1971.

periods of stimulation of the renal nerves in dogs produced practi-
cally identical increases in plasma renin activity (Figure 1).
However, if propranolol was administered before the second stimulation, the increase was abolished (Figure 2; see Assaykeen and
Ganong, 1971).

    We have also studied the effect of phenoxybenzamine on this
response.   In these experiments, phenoxybenzamine was administered
in a dose of 5 mg/kg, and mean blood pressure fell from 169/119
to 119/82 mmHg.   Associated with this decline in blood pressure
there was a marked increase in plasma renin activity before the
renal nerves were stimulated for the second time (Figure 3).   In
dogs given the same amount of phenoxybenzamine plus propranolol,
the hypotensive response was equally large but no rise in renin
secretion occurred.   Subsequent stimulation of the renal nerves
in the dogs given phenoxybenzamine alone produced an additional
rise in plasma renin activity, while no additional rise occurred
in the dogs that received phenoxybenzamine plus propranolol.   A
lack of effect of phenoxybenzamine on the renin response to renal
nerve stimulation has also been reported by Martin and White (1971).

    It seems likely that the increase in renin secretion produced
by phenoxybenzamine was secondary to the hypotension it produced.

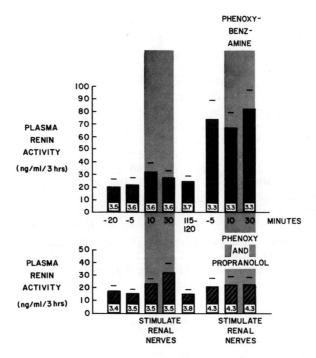

Figure 3.   Effect of phenoxybenzamine and of phenoxybenzamine
             plus propranolol on the increase in renin secretion
             produced by renal nerve stimulation in dogs. Renin
             measured by immunoassay. Values in bars are mean
             plasma potassium concentrations, in mEq/liter.

However, there is another possible explanation: phenoxybenzamine
decreased plasma potassium concentration, and such a decrease may
stimulate renin secretion (Vander, 1970). In the animals that
also received propranolol, mean plasma potassium actually rose,
due primarily to high values in one dog. However, the mean rise
was not statistically significant.

    Additional evidence for an intrarenal β-receptor affecting
renin secretion is the observation that the propranolol-blockable
increase in renin secretion produced by stimulation of the pressor
region of the medulla oblongata is blocked by sectioning the renal
nerves (Passo et al., 1970a, 1970b). This finding would be difficult to explain if the β-receptors involved were located outside
the kidneys.

    The increase in renin secretion produced by renal nerve stimu-
lation and infusions of catecholamines could of course be secondary to hemodynamic changes in the kidneys. However, Barajas (1964)

and others (for references see Assaykeen and Ganong, 1971) have
pointed out that there are many adrenergic nerves close to the
juxtaglomerular cells and some appear to make synaptic endings on
the secretory cells. Johnson et al. (1971) have recently reported
experiments in which stimulation of the renal nerves increased renin
secretion even when the glomerular filtration rate was apparently
zero and the renal baroreceptor mechanism "inactivated" by infusion
of the smooth muscle-relaxing agent, papaverine. They conclude from
these experiments that the increase in renin secretion is not mediated via the macula densa or the baroreceptor mechanism. Michelakis
and his associates (1969) have reported increased release of renin
from a renal cell suspension upon addition of epinephrine, norepinephrine, and cyclic AMP. Thus, although there is as yet no defini-
tive proof, it appears reasonable to suggest that the juxtaglomerular cells are neuroendocrine transducers with β receptors on their
cell membranes which respond directly to circulating catecholamines
or to norepinephrine liberated from adrenergic nerves in their vicinity. The evidence for intrarenal β receptors concerned with renin
secretion is summarized in Table II.

TABLE II

Evidence that the β-Receptor Affecting Renin Secretion
is in the Kidney

1. Stimulation of the renal nerves increases renin secretion.
    This response is:
    A. abolished by propranolol and unaffected by phenoxybenz-
          amine;
    B. present during infusion of papaverine;
    C. present during infusion of papaverine in the "nonfilter-
          ing kidney".
2. The propranolol-blockable increase in renin secretion pro-
    duced by stimulation of the brain stem is abolished by
    renal denervation.
3. Isoproterenol produces a greater increase in renin secretion
    when infused into the renal artery than when infused into a
    peripheral vein (Ayers).
4. Norepinephrine, epinephrine, and cyclic AMP stimulate renin
    release in vitro.
5. There are many adrenergic nerves among the juxtaglomerular
    cells, and there appear to be "en passant" synaptic junctions
    on the cells.

    It should be emphasized that the sympathetic nervous system
is only one of the mechanisms controlling renin secretion. Secretion also appears to be regulated by renal baroreceptors that
respond to afferent arteriolar pressure, the plasma concentration
of potassium and macula densa receptors that respond to sodium.

What role does the sympathetic nervous system play in the various
experimental and clinical conditions in which renin secretion is
increased? Its contribution can be assessed in two ways: its effect
can be blocked at the receptor level by administration of a β-
adrenergic blocking drug such as propranolol, or sympathetic outflow
can be interrupted. In experiments involving the latter approach,
it is important to section both the renal and adrenal nerves, since
both circulating epinephrine and norepinephrine released from the
endings of the renal nerves can affect renin secretion (Figure 4).

Stimuli that appear to be totally mediated by way of sympathetic activity include hypoglycemia and stimulation of the brain
stem. The former is blocked by propranolol and denervation of
the adrenal medulla, while the latter is blocked by propranolol
and section of the renal nerves. The increases in renin secretion produced by infusion of catecholamines and stimulation
of the renal nerves are also completely blocked by propranolol.

On the other hand, the increase in plasma renin activity
produced by pentobarbital anesthesia does not appear to be
sympathetically mediated. This rise is documented in Table III.

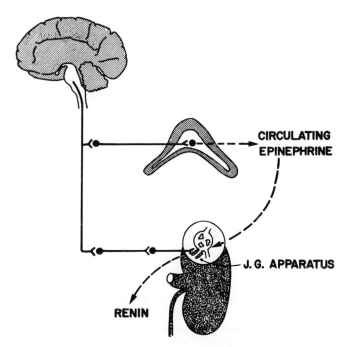

Figure 4.   Pathways by which the sympathetic nervous system
            can affect renin secretion. From Ganong, 1972.

TABLE III

Effect of Pentobarbital Anesthesia on
Plasma Renin Activity in Dogs

	Plasma renin activity (ng/ml, bioassay)
Unanesthetized (n=14)	4.0+0.7
Anesthetized (n=20)	10.0+2.3*

* p < 0.05

One might expect it to be due to increased sympathetic discharge
because cutting the renal nerves causes renal vasodilatation in
pentobarbital-anesthetized dogs (see Wise and Ganong, 1960).
However, as shown in Table IV, plasma renin activity is not
reduced after treatment with propranolol.

TABLE IV

Lack of Effect of Propranolol on Resting Plasma
Renin Levels in Pentobarbital Anesthetized Dogs*

	Plasma renin activity (ng/ml, bioassay)	
	Specimen 1	Specimen 2
No treatment (n=12)	8.1+1.1	9.4+1.7
Propranolol (n=6)	11.5+4.1	10.5+2.9

*Data are values in pre-insulin control periods
from Assaykeen et al., 1971.

The effect of adrenergic blockade on the renin response to
the diuretic furosemide has been studied by Mr. David MacDonald
in my laboratory. Confirming the results of others (see Vander
and Carlson, 1969), he has found that furosemide in a dose of
5 mg/kg intravenously produces a rapid rise in plasma renin activity upon injection into dogs in which volume loss is prevented by

connecting the ureters to the femoral veins. This increase is
unaffected by propranolol (Table V). Phenoxybenzamine produces
an increase in plasma renin activity before furosemide is administered, but furosemide still produces an additional increment in
plasma renin activity.

The role of the sympathetic nervous system in the increase in
renin secretion produced by adrenal insufficiency has been studied
by Dr. Harry Shizgal in my laboratory. He has followed plasma
renin levels during the development of adrenal insufficiency before and after renal denervation. Since the adrenals in these
animals were removed surgically, there was, of course, no adrenal
medulla to contend with. Plasma renin activity increased more
slowly in the dogs with denervated kidneys than in the controls,
but it eventually reached the same level (Figure 5).   In some
of these animals, plasma renin activity was determined by bioassay, while in the remainder it was determined by immunoassay.
However, when the animals are separated into two groups on the
basis of the assay used and analyzed separately, the results are
generally similar.

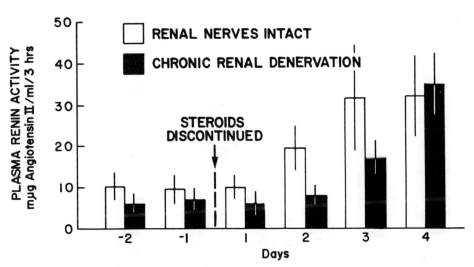

Figure 5.   Effect of renal denervation on the increase in plasma
renin activity produced by adrenal insufficiency.
Values are partly measured by bioassay and partly
by immunoassay.

TABLE V

Effect of Furosemide (5 mg/kg IV) on Plasma Renin Activity in Dogs
Treated with Propranolol* and Phenoxybenzamine**

Time (min before and after furosemide)	-5	5	15	30	60	120
No Treatment (n=14)	22.9+5.4	42.5+8.1	52.5+10.9	51.6+8.0	38.5+7.2	22.2+3.5
Propranolol (n=8)	22.8+7.8	38.3+10.5	42.7+11.1	52.9+12.0	41.2+8.2	23.1+5.6
Phenoxybenzamine (n=7)	63.1+15.2	86.6+19.2	88.0+18.5	81.0+16.0	78.6+19.6	66.0+14.7

*0.6 mg/kg followed by 0.3 mg/kg/hour intravenously
**5 mg/kg intravenously

Shizgal also gave propranolol to anesthetized adrenally insufficient dogs and followed their plasma renin activity. The renins were again measured in part by bioassay and in part by immunoassay. The bioassay results were erratic, while the immunoassay results showed a decline in plasma renin activity during the propranolol infusion. Thus, no conclusion is possible at present and additional studies are being carried out to settle the point. However, it appears that the increase in plasma renin activity produced by adrenal insufficiency is mediated in part by way of the sympathetic nervous system, but that other mechanisms are also involved.

The role of the sympathetic nervous system in the increase in renin secretion produced by a low sodium diet has been studied by Vander and his associates. In humans with transplanted kidneys, the renin response to dietary sodium restriction was found to be normal (Green and Vander, 1968; Blaufox et al., 1969), but circulating catecholamines were not measured in these studies and re-innervation of the transplants was not excluded. Brubacher and Vander (1968) found that bilateral renal denervation in dogs slowed the renin response to dietary sodium restriction; during the first three days of the low sodium diet, the denervated animals had lower plasma renins, but by the fourth day the renin level in the controls and the denervated dogs was equal. It is of interest in this regard that feeding dogs a low sodium diet for 14 days does not cause any measurable increase in plasma catecholamines (Table VI). Our control diet provides approximate 40 mEq of sodium per day, while our low sodium diet provides less than 1 mEq per day.

TABLE VI

Effect of Dietary Sodium Restriction on Plasma
Epinephrine and Norepinephrine

Arterial Plasma Catecholamines* (ng/ml)

		Epinephrine	Norepinephrine	
Control Diet	Day 1	0.7+0.2	1.4+0.4	(4)
	2	0.4+0.2	1.2+0.3	(4)
	3	0.3+0.1	0.9+0.3	(5)
Low Sodium Diet	Day 5	0.4+0.1	1.2+0.1	(4)
	14	0.4+0.2	1.1+0.2	(6)

*Method of Goldfien, A., S.Zileli, D. Goodman, and G.W. Thorn, The estimation of epinephrine and norepinephrine in human plasma. J Clin Endocr Metab 21:281-295, 1961.

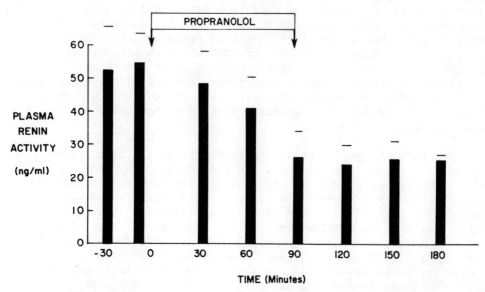

Figure 6.   Effect of propranolol on plasma renin activity in
            dogs that had been fed a low sodium diet for two
            weeks, then anesthetized with pentobarbital. Renin
            measured by immunoassay. Propranolol was infused
            intravenously in a dose of 0.6 mg/kg, followed by a
            constant infusion of 0.3 mg/kg/hour.

        Brubacher and Vander (1968) also reported that acute infu-
sions of phenoxybenzamine and propranolol had no greater effect
on plasma renin activity than saline in dogs fed a low sodium
diet. We placed 6 dogs on a low sodium diet for two weeks, then
anesthetized them with pentobarbital and infused propranolol while
following changes in plasma renin activity. The results are shown
in Figure 6.

The decrease in plasma renin activity was statistically significant. We anesthetized three dogs that had been fed a normal
sodium diet and followed their plasma renin activity at half-hour
intervals throughout the day. The levels were stable except for
an unexplained transient increase during the fourth hour in one
of the dogs. To determine if propranolol also reduced levels in
anesthetized dogs regardless of sodium intake, three dogs fed a
normal sodium diet were infused with propranolol. The renin
levels in these dogs, which were low to start with, did not change
(Figure 7). However, there remained the possibility that the
high initial renin level in anesthetized dogs fed a low sodium
diet would decline spontaneously without administration of

propranolol. This possibility has been explored in two dogs, and the data are inconclusive. More animals will have to be studied before any firm conclusion can be drawn.

Thus, it appears likely that the sympathetic nervous system does contribute to the increase in renin secretion produced by a low sodium diet. However, other factors are also involved, and when the sodium deficiency becomes marked, these mechanisms can compensate for the absence of the sympathetic component.

In conclusion, the bulk of the available evidence indicates that the sympathetic nervous system can stimulate renin secretion by way of β-adrenergic receptors, and there is reason to believe these receptors are located on the juxtaglomerular cells. The contribution of the sympathetic nervous system to increased renin secretion varies with the stimulus. The data on this contribution are summarized in Table VII. The sympathetic nervous system is the major mediator of the increases produced by hypoglycemia, stimulation of the medulla oblongata and phenoxybenzamine. It

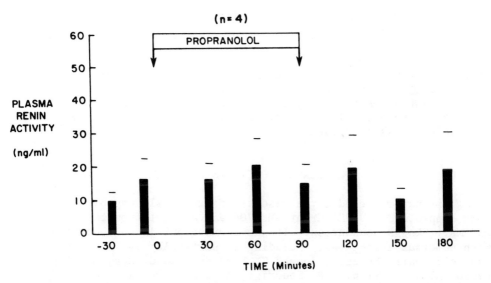

Figure 7. Effect of propranolol on plasma renin activity in dogs that had been fed a normal sodium diet and then anesthetized with pentobarbital. Renin determined by immunoassay. The propranolol was infused intravenously in a dose of 0.6 mg/kg, followed by a constant infusion of 0.3 mg/kg/hour.

TABLE VII

Effect of Sympathetic Blockade on the Increase in
Renin Secretion Produced by Various Stimuli

	Interrupt Sympathetic Outflow	Propranolol
Hypoglycemia	block by adrenal nerve section	block
Stimulate medulla oblongata	block by renal nerve section	block
Epinephrine, isoproterenol	-	block
Stimulate renal nerves	-	block
Pentobarbital anesthesia	-	no block
Furosemide	-	no block
Adrenal insufficiency	partial block	?
Low sodium diet	partial block	?

appears to contribute to the response to a low sodium diet and
adrenal insufficiency, but with time other mechanisms can compensate for its absence. It apparently plays no role in the response to pentobarbital anesthesia and to the diuretic furosemide
when volume loss is prevented.

ACKNOWLEDGEMENTS

    This paper includes the results of previously unpublished
work supproted by USPHS Grant AM06704 and a grant from the L.J.
and Mary Skaggs Foundation. It was carried out in collaboration
with numerous associates, including in particular Tania Assaykeen,
Ian Reid, Harry Shizgal, Thomas C. Lee, Kensaku Otsuka, Stanley
Passo, Alan Goldfien, J.R. Stockigt, Angela Boryczka, John
Loeffler, Roy Shackelford, and David MacDonald.

REFERENCES

Allison, D.J., P.L. Clayton, S.S. Passo, and T.A. Assaykeen,
    The effect of isoproterenol and adrenergic blocking agents
    on plasma renin activity and renal function in anesthetized
    dogs, Fed Proc 29:782, 1970 (abstract).

Assaykeen, T.A. and W.F. Ganong, The sympathetic nervous system
    and renin secretion. In:Frontiers in Neuroendocrinology,
    1971, L. Martini and W.F. Ganong, eds., pp. 67-102, Oxford
    University Press, New York, 1971.

Assaykeen, T.A., P.L. Clayton, A. Goldfien, and W.F. Ganong,
    The effect of α- and β-adrenergic blocking agents on the
    renin response to hypoglycemia and epinephrine in dogs,
    Endocrinology 87:1318-1322, 1970.

Ayers, C.R., R.H. Harris, Jr., and L.G. Lefer, Control of renin
    release in experimental hypertension, Circ Res 24: Suppl I,
    103-112, 1969.

Barajas, L., The innervation of the juxtaglomerular apparatus,
    Lab Invest 13:916-929, 1964.

Blaufox, M.D., E.J. Lewis, P. Jagger, D. Lauler, R. Hickler, and
    J.P. Merrill, Physiologic responses of the transplanted
    human kidney, New England J Med 280:62-66, 1969.

Brubacher, E.S. and A.J. Vander, Sodium deprivation and renin
    secretion in unanesthetized dogs, Am J Physiol 214:15-21,
    1968.

Ganong, W.F., Pharmacological aspects of neuroendocrine integra-
    tion. Progress in Brain Research, in press, 1972.

Greene, J.A., Jr., and A.J. Vander, Plasma renin activity and
    aldosterone excretion after renal homotransplantation,
    J Lab Clin Med 71:586-595, 1968.

Gump, F.E., T. Magill, A.P. Thal, and J.M. Kinney, Regional
    adrenergic blockade by intra-arterial injection of phenoxy-
    benzamine, Surg Gynec Obst 127:319-326, 1968.

Johnson, J.A., J.O. Davis, and R.T. Witty, Control of renin
    secretion by the renal sympathetic nerves, The Physiologist
    14:168, 1971 (abstract).

Martin, D.M. and F.N. White, Evidence for direct neural release
    of renin, Fed Proc 30:431, 1971 (abstract).

Michelakis, A.M., J. Caudle, and D.W. Liddle, In vitro stimula-
    tion of renin production by epinephrine, norepinephrine,
    and cyclic AMP, Proc Soc Exp Biol Med 130:748-753, 1969.

Otsuka, K., T.A. Assaykeen, A. Goldfien, and W.F. Ganong, The
    effect of hypoglycemia on plasma renin activity in dogs,
    Endocrinology 87:1306-1317, 1970.

Passo, S.S., T.A. Assaykeen, K. Otsuka, B.L. Wise, A. Goldfien,
    and W.F. Ganong, Effect of stimulation of the medulla
    oblongata on renin secretion in dogs, Neuroendocrinology
    7:1-10, 1971a.

Passo, S.S., T.A. Assaykeen, A. Goldfien, and W.F. Ganong, Effect
    of α- and β-adrenergic blocking agents on the increase in

renin secretion produced by stimulation of the medulla oblongata in dogs, Neuroendocrinology 7:94-104, 1971b.

Reid, I.A. and W.F. Ganong, Effect of theophylline on renin secretion, Fed. Proc. 30:449, 1971 (abstract).

Robison, G.A. and E.W. Sutherland, Sympathin E, sympathin I, and the intracellular level of cyclic AMP, Circ. Res. 26: Suppl I, 147-162, 1970.

Ueda, H., H. Yasuda, Y. Takabatake, M. Iizuka, T. Iizuka, M. Ihori, and Y. Sakamoto, Observations on the mechanism of renin release by catecholamines, Circ. Res. 26: Suppl II, 195-200, 1970.

Vander, A.J., Direct effects of potassium on renin secretion and renal function, Am. J. Physiol. 219:455-459, 1970.

Vander, A.J. and J. Carlson, Mechanism of the effects of furosemide on renin secretion in anesthetized dogs, Circ. Res. 25:145-152, 1969.

Winer, N., B.H. Burch, D.S. Chokshi, and A.D. Freedman, Cyclic AMP stimulation of renin secretion, Program of the 51st Meeting of the Endocrine Society, New York, p. 100, 1969 (abstract).

Wise, B.L. and W.F. Ganong, Effect of brain stem stimulation on renal function, Am. J. Physiol. 198:1291-1295, 1960.

THE EFFECTS OF CYCLIC NUCLEOTIDES ON PLASMA RENIN ACTIVITY AND

RENAL FUNCTION IN DOGS.

D. J. Allison, H. Tanigawa and T.A. Assaykeen

Departments of Surgery (Urology) and Pharmacology,

Stanford University School of Medicine, Stanford,

California

It has been reported previously by our laboratory (Allison et al.,1970) that isoproterenol infused into the renal artery resulted in a significant increase in plasma renin activity in the absence of significant changes in blood pressure, plasma potassium concentration or renal function. Beta adrenergic blockade was effective in preventing the increase in plasma renin activity associated with isoproterenol infusion, whereas alpha adrenergic blockade was without effect.

Robison et al. (1968) have shown that beta adrenergic blocking agents act as competitive inhibitors in adenyl cyclase systems activated by catecholamines. It has also been suggested that adenyl cyclase is part of the beta adrenergic receptor (Robison et al., 1967). Therefore it was thought that a direct effect of isoproterenol on renin secretion might be mediated via increased activity of adenyl cyclase in renin-secreting cells. If this is true, it should be possible to mimic the effects of beta adrenergic stimulation by administration of cyclic AMP, the product of adenyl cyclase. In support of this assumption, Winer et al. (1969a) reported that infusion of cyclic AMP (0.3 mg/min) into the renal artery of dogs resulted in an increase in renal venous renin activity within 30 minutes. On the other hand, Tagawa and Vander (1970) observed no increase in renin secretion when cyclic AMP at 1.0-5.0 mg/min was infused into the renal artery of sodium deplete dogs.

Theophylline is capable of mimicking cyclic AMP effects in certain systems, probably by inhibiting degradation of the nucleotide by phosphodiesterase (Butcher and Sutherland, 1962). In man,

33

theophylline infusion has been associated with an increase in
plasma renin activity (Winer et al., 1969b). Recently, Reid and
Ganong (1971) have shown that infusion of theophylline into dogs
also is associated with an increase in plasma renin activity.
These experiments add support to the idea that the adenyl cyclase
system plays a role in renin secretion.

The studies to be presented were performed to add evidence to
that described above. The effect on plasma renin activity of intrarenal infusions of 5'-AMP, cyclic AMP and dibutyryl cyclic AMP was
studied in normal and sodium deplete dogs, alone and in the presence
of theophylline (Section A). The 5'-AMP was employed as a control
substance. Dibutyryl cyclic AMP was used because it apparently
penetrates cell membranes more readily and is more resistant to
breakdown by phosphodiesterase than is cyclic AMP itself (Posternak
et al., 1962). In Section B, theophylline was administered into
the renal artery of sodium deplete dogs at 2.5 mg/min, the same
dose used in conjunction with certain of the nucleotide infusions
in Section A. These experiments were designed to study the effects
on plasma renin activity of this dosage of theophylline alone. And
finally, Section C describes experiments in which dibutyryl cyclic
AMP plus theophylline was administered to sodium deplete dogs in
order to assess the simultaneous effects of this drug combination
on renal function and plasma renin activity.

MATERIALS AND METHODS

Experimental Animals. Experiments were performed on 27 male
mongrel dogs weighing 11-18 kg (Section A), 11-14 kg (Section B)
and 9-16 kg (Section C). Twelve dogs in Section A were maintained
on a normal laboratory diet. The remaining 15 dogs were fed a
liquid low-sodium diet (Lonalac, Mead Johnson Labs; less than 1 mEq
Na/day) for 7 days prior to the experiment. All dogs were fasted
overnight before the experiment, but were allowed free access to
water. Anesthesia was induced with pentobarbital sodium (30 mg/kg)
with supplements being administered as required.

Surgical Procedures. The left femoral artery was cannulated
for withdrawal of blood samples and continuous monitoring of blood
pressure via a Statham strain gauge connected to a Model 7 Grass
polygraph. A left femoral vein cannula was the route for anesthesia
supplements and whole blood replacement. Through a right flank incision, a left nephrectomy was performed. A fish-hook-shaped modified scalp vein needle was inserted into the right renal artery.
Patency of the needle was maintained by infusion of 5% dextrose in
water plus 1% heparin at a rate of 0.24 ml/min. Handling of the
kidney and dissection of the renal pedicle were minimal. In experiments where function studies were performed (Section C), the right

ureter was cannulated and an indwelling catheter was placed into a foreleg vein for infusion of PAH and inulin.

Experimental Protocols. Section A (n=16). At least one and one-half hours after completion of surgery, the experiment was started. Ten ml samples of arterial blood were collected in heparin for measurement of sodium and potassium. Femoral arterial blood (30 ml samples) was also collected into a tube containing 3.8% EDTA (ammonium form, pH 6.5, 1 ml/10 ml of blood) for measurement of plasma renin activity. All blood withdrawn was replaced with whole blood from a nephrectomized donor dog. Following collection of control blood samples, an infusion of one of the three nucleotides in 5% dextrose in water plus 1% heparin was started into the renal artery at a rate of 0.24 ml/min. The nucleotides used were: 5'-AMP (adenosine-5'-monophosphate, Calbiochem), cyclic AMP (cAMP, adenosine 3',5'-cyclic monophosphate, Calbiochem) and dibutyryl cyclic AMP (DBcAMP, N^6, 0^2 -dibutyryl adenosine-3',5'-cyclic phosphate, Calbiochem). These compounds were infused at doses equivalent on a molar basis to 0.3, 1.0 and 2.5 mg cAMP/min. In a few experiments, as indicated in the Results Section, theophylline (equivalent weight to that of the nucleotide, Mann Research Laboratories) was infused with the nucleotide. In some of the experiments, the pH of the nucleotide solution was adjusted to 7.4 with NaOH before use, as indicated in the Results Section. Fifteen and 30 minutes following the start of the nucleotide infusion, blood samples were again collected. The nucleotide infusion was then discontinued and a 30 minute period allowed to elapse before collection of the next set of control blood samples and the start of the next nucleotide infusion. Each animal received all three nucleotides. The usual order of nucleotide administration was : 5'-AMP, cAMP and DBcAMP since the renin rise seen following DBcAMP infusion was prolonged. In some of the experiments at the highest dosage level, an additional blood sample was taken 30 minutes after discontinuation of the DBcAMP infusion.

Section B (n=5). The experimental protocol for animals in this group was identical to that described for Section A except for the omission of nucleotides from the infusion solution. Thus each animal received 3, 30 minute infusions of theophylline (2.5 mg/min), each separated by a 30 minute control period. An additional set of blood samples were taken 30 minutes after completion of the third theophylline infusion. Renin was measured by immunoassay (see below) and thus required the removal of only 10 ml of blood for this measurement at each sampling period.

Section C (n=6). At the completion of surgery a saline infusion was begun at 0.24 ml/min into a peripheral vein. Following equilibration of the urine flow at a minimal level of 0.1 ml/min, and at least one and one-half hours after completion of surgery, a plasma sample was withdrawn as a blank for subsequent PAH and inulin

TABLE I

Effects of Infusion of 5'-AMP into the Renal Artery of Dogs

Time min	Dose	Plasma Renin Activity mµg/ml/3hr	Blood Pressure mm Hg Systolic	Diastolic	Plasma Electrolytes mEq/L Sodium	Potassium
	0.3 mg/min					
0	(n=3)	21.2 ±12.8	165 ± 10	113 ± 9	149 ± 3	3.9 ± 0.1
+15		13.1 ± 8.0	168 ± 9	118 ± 7	150 ± 2	3.7 ± 0.2
+30		10.8 ± 6.1	167 ± 11	118 ± 7	151 ± 2	3.5 ± 0.2*
	1.0 mg/min					
0	(n=4)	14.2 ± 3.9	158 ± 9	120 ±11	146 ± 1	3.9 ± 0.3
+15		10.0 ± 2.5	159 ± 11	115 ± 9	147 ± 1	3.8 ± 0.4
+30		11.4 ± 2.6	158 ± 13	119 ±11	148 ± 1	3.7 ± 0.4
	2.5 mg/min					
0	(n=6)	16.3 ± 3.1	164 ± 8	114 ± 6	146 ± 1	4.1 ± 0.2
+15		14.3 ± 2.5	161 ± 8	111 ± 5	147 ± 1	4.0 ± 0.2
+30		14.4 ± 2.1	158 ± 9	109 ± 7	148 ± 1	3.9 ± 0.2*
	1.0 mg/min plus 2.5 mg/min					
0	(n=10)	15.4 ± 2.3	162 ± 6	117 ± 5	146 ± 1	4.0 ± 0.1
+15		12.6 ± 1.9*	160 ± 6	113 ± 4	147 ± 1	3.9 ± 0.2*
+30		13.2 ± 1.6	158 ± 7	113 ± 6	148 ± 1*	3.8 ± 0.2**

Data expressed as means ± one standard error.
* $p < 0.05$ when compared to the respective 0 minute control value.
**$p < 0.01$ when compared to the respective 0 minute control value.

determinations. Priming doses of PAH (sodium aminohippurate, Merck, Sharpe and Dome) and inulin (Arnar-Stone Labs., Inc.) were then administered intravenously, followed by a continuous infusion of PAH and inulin in normal saline at 0.24 ml/min. The priming and maintenance doses were calculated for each dog and were designed to maintain plasma concentrations of PAH and inulin at 2 and 20 mg/100 ml blood, respectively. Twenty-five minutes later, a control clearance period was performed. Throughout the experiment, the duration of the clearance periods averaged 15 minutes. Urine samples obtained were measured for volume and sodium, potassium, PAH and inulin concentrations. Samples of arterial blood were collected as described in Section B at the midpoint of each clearance period. In this series each dog received an intrarenal infusion of DBcAMP(3.75 mg/min - equivalent on a molar basis to 2.5 mg cAMP/min) plus theophylline (2.5 mg/min) for 30 minutes and an additional set of blood samples was withdrawn 30 minutes after the infusion was stopped.

Analytical Techniques. Standard clearance techniques were used
to determine the glomerular filtration rate (GFR; inulin clearance)
and effective renal plasma flow (RPF; PAH clearance). Inulin was
measured by the method of Hagashi and Peters (1950) as modified by
Fjeldbo and Stamey (1968); PAH was determined as described by
Harvey and Brothers (1962). The products of both reactions were
determined spectrophotometrically on a Technicon AutoAnalyzer.
Plasma renin activity in the experiments in Section A was measured
by the method of Boucher et al. (1964) with slight modifications as
previously described (Assaykeen et al., 1968). In Sections B and C,
plasma renin activity was measured by radioimmunoassay of angiotensin
I (Stockigt et al., 1971). With both methods, plasma renin activity
(PRA) is expressed as mµg angiotensin generated/ml of plasma/3 hours
of incubation. Plasma and urinary electrolytes were determined by

TABLE II

Effects of Infusion of Cyclic AMP into the
Renal Artery of Dogs

Time min	Dose	Plasma Renin Activity	Blood Pressure mm Hg		Plasma Electrolytes mEq/L	
		mµg/ml/3hr	Systolic	Diastolic	Sodium	Potassium
	0.3 mg/min					
0	(n=6)	15.4 ± 4.8	170 ± 8	118 ± 6	148 ± 1	3.7 ± 0.1
+15		15.2 ± 5.4	172 ± 7	123 ± 5	148 ± 1	3.6 ± 0.1
+30		13.1 ± 4.2	173 ± 6	120 ± 4	149 ± 1	3.6 ± 0.1
	1.0 mg/min					
0	(n=4)	7.9 ± 2.6	164 ± 10	111 ± 5	147 ± 1	3.9 ± 0.4
+15		7.7 ± 1.9	165 ± 11	124 ±11	147 ± 1	4.1 ± 0.3
+30		8.2 ± 2.1	161 ± 10	119 ± 9	148 ± 1	4.0 ± 0.3
	2.5 mg/min					
0	(n=6)	15.1 ± 2.4	163 + 8	114 ± 6	148 ± 1	4.0 ± 0.2
+15		15.0 ± 2.2	168 ± 8*	118 ± 4	148 ± 1	4.0 ± 0.2
+30		17.0 ± 4.5	162 ± 8	114 ± 5	149 ± 1*	3.9 ± 0.2
	1.0 mg/min plus 2.5 mg/min					
0	(n=10)	12.2 ± 2.0	163 ± 6	113 ± 4	147 ± 1	4.0 ± 0.2
+15		12.1 ± 1.9	167 ± 6*	120 ± 5	148 ± 1	4.1 ± 0.2
+30		13.5 ± 3.0	162 ± 6	116 ± 4	148 ± 1*	3.9 ± 0.2

Data expressed as means ± one standard error.
* $p < 0.05$ when compared with the respective 0 min control value.

TABLE III

Effects of Infusion of Dibutyryl Cyclic AMP into
the Renal Artery of Dogs

Time min	Dose	Plasma Renin Activity	Blood Pressure mm Hg		Plasma Electrolytes mEq/L	
		mµg/ml/3hr	Systolic	Diastolic	Sodium	Potassium
	0.3 mg/min					
0	(n=3)	9.0 ± 4.0	173 ± 4	127 ± 3	145 ± 1	3.7 ± 0.1
+15		9.3 ± 4.4	175 ± 5	130 ± 3	145 ± 1	3.6 ± 0.1
+30		9.6 ± 5.2	175 ± 3	133 ± 2	146 ± 1	3.4 ± 0.2
	1.0 mg/min					
0	(n=4)	8.1 ± 1.3	161 ± 12	124 ±11	148 ± 1	4.1 ± 0.4
+15		9.1 ± 1.6	160 ± 12	124 ±11	148 ± 1	4.1 ± 0.4
+30		9.8 ± 1.4	159 ± 12	121 ±12	148 ± 1	3.7 ± 0.4
	2.5 mg/min					
0	(n=6)	20.6 ± 4.5	163 ± 6	117 ± 4	149 ± 1	3.9 ± 0.2
+15		20.1 ± 4.0	163 ± 8	118 ± 4	149 ± 1	3.9 ± 0.2
+30		28.6 ± 5.4	168 ± 10	120 ± 4	149 ± 1	3.7 ± 0.1
+60†		37.9 ± 7.6*	166 ± 9	118 ± 3	150 ± 1	3.7 ± 0.2
	1.0 mg/min plus 2.5 mg/min					
0	(n=10)	15.6 ± 3.3	163 ± 6	120 ± 5	148 ± 1	4.0 ± 0.2
+15		15.7 ± 3.0	162 ± 6	121 ± 5	149 ± 1	4.0 ± 0.2
+30		21.1 ± 4.4	164 ± 7	121 ± 5	149 ± 1	3.7 ± 0.2*
+60†		30.8 ± 7.3*	167 ± 8	120 ± 6	149 ± 2	3.7 ± 0.2*

Data expressed as means ± one standard error.
* p < 0.05 when compared to the respective 0 min control value.
† 30 minutes after DBcAMP infusion was stopped.

flame photometry. Hematocrit was determined by the microcapillary
tube method. Filtration fraction (FF) was calculated as C_{inulin}/C_{PAH}. Statistical analysis of the difference between control and
experimental periods was determined by use of the t-test on paired
observations (Goldstein, 1964).

RESULTS

Section A. The results obtained for all variables studied are
shown in Tables I (5'-AMP), II (cAMP) and III (DBcAMP).

When 5'-AMP was infused into the renal artery of dogs, no statistically significant changes in PRA were observed with any of the 3 dosage levels used; rather, 5'-AMP infusion appeared to be associated with a decrease in PRA. When data from the 2 higher dosage levels were pooled and analyzed together (n=10), the decrease in PRA was statistically significant ($p < 0.05$) at the 15 minute experimental period. The left hand panel of Figure 1 gives PRA changes for the individual dogs at these dosage levels. Each line represents the values from a single dog. Adjustment of the pH of the infusion, administration of theophylline or prior low-salt diet did not appear to alter the response to 5'-AMP infusion.

As observed with 5'-AMP, cAMP infusion into the renal artery was not associated with any significant changes in PRA. At 0.3 mg/min, PRA levels decreased slightly in all of the 6 animals studied. The center panel of Figure 1 presents PRA levels in individual dogs during cAMP infusion at the 2 higher dosage levels. At 1 mg/min, PRA levels increased slightly in 2, decreased in 1 and showed no

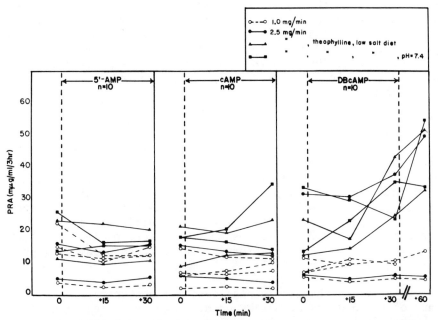

Figure 1.   PRA in individual dogs during 5'-AMP, cyclic AMP and dibutyryl cyclic AMP infusions (1.0 and 2.5 mg/min) into the renal artery. Each line represents the response of a single animal to infusions of 5'-AMP (left panel), cAMP (center panel) and DBcAMP (right panel). The dashed lines indicate a dose of 1.0 mg/min; the solid lines represent a dose of 2.5 mg/min. Different symbols represent changes in experimental protocol as summarized in the box in the upper right hand corner.

change in 1 dog. At 2.5 mg/min, PRA levels decreased in 3 of the
6 animals. In the other 3 animals, where PRA levels increased
during cAMP infusion, low-salt diet and concurrent theophylline infusion were included in the protocol. In 2 of the 3 animals, the
pH of the infusing solution had previously been adjusted to 7.4 with
NaOH.

    With infusion of 0.3 mg/min DBcAMP, an increase in PRA was seen
in 1 of the 3 dogs studied. In the right hand panel of Figure 1 are
presented the PRA values from individual dogs at the two higher
doses. At a dose of 1.0 mg/min, increases in PRA were seen in 3 of
4 experiments. However, no significant changes in mean values were
observed. At this dosage it was noted that, in 2 animals from which
blood samples were obtained, a delayed increase in PRA could be
observed 30 minutes following discontinuation of DBcAMP infusion.
Therefore, at the highest dosage such an additional sample was taken
in all animals and is labelled as the 60 minute experimental period
in Table III and Figure I. An increase in PRA levels occurred in 5
of 6 animals studied at this dosage level. This change was significant ($p < 0.05$) at the 60 minute sampling period. Four of these
animals had received a low-sodium diet plus concurrent theophylline
infusion. In 3 of these animals, the pH of the infusion solution
had previously been adjusted to 7.4 with NaOH. When the data for
the 2 higher dosage levels were pooled and analyzed together, a significant increase in PRA ($p < 0.05$) was again noted at the 60 minute
experimental period.

    No statistically significant changes in mean systolic or dia-
stolic blood pressure were associated with 5'-AMP or DBcAMP infusions
into the renal artery at any of the 3 dosage levels. During cAMP
infusion at the 2 lower dosage levels, there were also no significant
changes in mean systolic or diastolic pressure. However, at a dose
of 2.5 mg/min, both systolic and diastolic blood pressures were increased slightly at the 15 minute experimental period; the change in
systolic blood pressure was statistically significant ($p < 0.05$).
When the data for the 2 higher dosage levels were pooled (n=10), the
increase in systolic blood pressure at the 15 minute sampling period
was also significant ($p < 0.05$).

    No significant changes in plasma sodium concentration were seen
with any of the 3 doses of 5'-AMP used. However, when the data for
the 2 higher dosage levels were pooled and analyzed together (n=10),
the slight rise in plasma sodium concentration seen at the 30 minute
experimental period was statistically significant ($p < 0.05$). At the
two lower dosage levels of cAMP, the plasma sodium concentration
showed no significant changes. At a dose of 2.5 mg/min, the small
increase seen in plasma sodium concentration was statistically significant ($p < 0.05$) at the 30 minute experimental period. When data
from the 2 higher dosage levels were pooled (n=10), the increase in

TABLE IV

Effects of Infusion of Theophylline (2.5 mg/min)
into the Renal Artery of Dogs (n=5)

Time	Plasma Renin Activity	Blood Pressure Systolic	Diastolic	Plasma Electrolytes Sodium	Potassium
(min)	(mμg/ml/3hr)	(mm Hg)		(mEq/L)	
0	36.8 ± 7.5	166 ± 11	114 ± 7	142 ± 2	3.6 ± 0.2
+15	56.2 ± 13.9*	166 ± 7	112 ± 6	142 ± 2	3.6 ± 0.2
+30	62.3 ± 16.0	153 ± 10	107 ± 6	143 ± 2	3.6 ± 0.2
0	53.6 ± 16.3	151 ± 10	107 ± 7	143 ± 3	3.5 ± 0.2
+15	73.7 ± 22.0	156 ± 12	109 ± 8	144 ± 3	3.6 ± 0.2
+30	76.5 ± 20.0*	153 ± 12	105 ± 7	144 ± 3	3.5 ± 0.2
0	68.9 ± 23.0	147 ± 12	103 ± 9	145 ± 3	3.4 ± 0.1
+15	77.3 ± 23.7	149 ± 10	103 ± 8	145 ± 3	3.3 ± 0.2
+30	77.1 ± 26.0	147 ± 10	104 ± 8	146 ± 3	3.5 ± 0.2
+60†	71.1 ± 25.9	145 ± 11	102 ±11	145 ± 3	3.4 ± 0.3

Data expressed as mean ± one standard error.
* $p < 0.05$ when compared to the respective 0 min control value.
† 30 minutes after infusion of theophylline was stopped.

plasma sodium concentration at the 30 minute sampling period was
also significant ($p < 0.05$). Plasma sodium concentration did not
change significantly from the control levels during DBcAMP infusion
at any of the 3 dosage levels used.

Plasma potassium concentration decreased following the infusion
of 5'-AMP into the renal artery at each of the 3 doses employed.
This decrease was statistically significant ($p < 0.05$) at the 30
minute experimental period with infusion of 0.3 or 2.5 mg/min. When
the data for 1.0 and 2.5 mg/min were analyzed together (n=10), the
decrease in plasma potassium concentration was significant at the
15 ($p < 0.05$) and 30 minute ($p < 0.01$) sampling periods. During
the infusion of cAMP, plasma potassium concentration showed no
significant changes from the control level at any of the 3 dosage
levels used. Plasma potassium concentration decreased slightly
during DBcAMP infusion at each of the dosage levels. When data for
the two higher dosage levels were pooled (n=10), the decrease in
plasma potassium concentration was statistically significant ($p <
0.05$) at the 30 and 60 minute experimental periods.

Section B.   Table IV shows the results obtained for all variables studied during infusion of theophylline (2.5 mg/min) into the
renal artery of 5 sodium deplete dogs.

PRA rose significantly during the first 2 experimental periods.
During the first experimental period, PRA was increased above the
initial control level after 15 minutes of infusion (p < 0.05).
During the second experimental period the increase in PRA above both
the initial control value and the corresponding 0 minute control
level was significant (p < 0.05) at the 30 minute time period.   No
significant change in PRA from either the initial value or the
corresponding control level was observed during the third and last
experimental period.   There appeared to be a gradual rise in the
control PRA level in each of the 5 animals from the first infusion
of theophylline to the third but this difference was not statistically significant, probably because of the large standard errors.

No significant changes in mean systolic or diastolic blood
pressure or in plasma sodium and potassium concentration were observed following theophylline infusion at any of the sampling times within the 3 experimental periods.

Section C.   Table V shows the results obtained for all variables
studied during the intrarenal infusion of DBcAMP plus theophylline
in this series of experiments.

PRA rose in 5 out of 6 dogs within 30 minutes and remained
elevated in 4 of these animals 30 minutes after the infusion was
stopped.   The 6th animal had a very high PRA at the control sampling
period which decreased during the first 15 minutes of infusion and
then rose steadily during the remainder of the experiment.

During the infusion of DBcAMP plus theophylline there were no
significant changes in systolic or diastolic blood pressure or in
plasma sodium concentration.   Plasma potassium concentration, however, decreased significantly at both the 30 and 60 minute experimental periods (p < 0.01).

Marked changes in renal function occurred during infusion of
DBcAMP and theophylline.   There were statistically significant rises
in urinary sodium and potassium excretion within 15 minutes.   These
significant changes persisted for up to 30 minutes after the infusion was stopped and were accompanied by corresponding rises in urinary volume.   GFR and RPF rose slightly but significantly at the 15
minute sampling period without a corresponding change in filtration
fraction.   No other significant changes were seen in these three
variables.   In spite of the large losses in sodium and water, there
were no significant changes in hematocrit throughout the experiment.

TABLE V

Effects of Infusion of DBcAMP Plus Theophylline into
the Renal Artery of Sodium Deplete Dogs (n=6)

	Control	+15 min	+30 min	+60 min†
PRA (mμg/ml/3hr)	85.5 ± 21.4	82.4 ± 20.9	120.2 ± 22.9	110.8 ± 15.0
BP systolic	165 ± 6	164 ± 7	166 ± 9	160 ± 11
diastolic (mm Hg)	114 ± 4	113 ± 4	111 ± 5	110 ± 7
Plasma [Na]	141 ± 2	141 ± 2	140 ± 2	142 ± 2
[K] (mEq/L)	3.5 ± 0.2	3.6 ± 0.2	3.3 ± 0.2**	3.1 ± 0.3**
Urinary Na	12 ± 3	72 ± 21*	160 ± 50*	155 ± 55*
K (μEq/min)	18 ± 3	33 ± 6**	40 ± 8**	34 ± 8*
Urine Flow (ml/min)	0.3 ± 0.1	1.0 ± 0.2*	2.0 ± 0.5*	1.8 ± 0.6
GFR (ml/min/kg)	1.7 ± 0.2	2.1 ± 0.2*	1.8 ± 0.1	1.6 ± 0.2
RPF (ml/min/kg)	5.3 ± 0.7	6.3 ± 0.7*	6.3 ± 0.3	4.9 ± 0.4
FF (%)	32 ± 3	34 ± 2	29 ± 2	33 ± 3
Hematocrit (%)	37 ± 2	37 ± 2	37 ± 2	38 ± 2

Data expressed as mean ± one standard error.
* $p < 0.05$ when compared to the control value.
** $p < 0.01$ when compared to the control value
† 30 minutes after infusion of DBcAMP plus theophylline was stopped.

DISCUSSION

The data presented in Section A indicate that at the doses
used, only DBcAMP and not 5'-AMP and cAMP was associated with an
increase in PRA. A similar lack of effect of 5'-AMP on renin secretion in dogs was noted by both Winer et al. (1969a) and Tagawa and
Vander (1970). Our results with the infusion of cAMP (0.3 - 2.5
mg/min) also agree with the results of Tagawa and Vander (1970) who
observed no increase in renin secretion with infusions of 1.0 - 5.0
mg/min of this nucleotide. Our results are at variance, however,
with those of Winer et al. (1969a) who showed an increase in renin
secretion within 30 minutes after starting an infusion of 0.3 mg/min
cAMP into the renal artery of dogs. An explanation for this dis-
crepancy is not possible. Michelakis et al. (1969) also demonstrated an effect of cAMP on renin in a renal cell suspension system. In
their in vitro system, however, cAMP may have had more ready access
into the cells, and thus have been able to exert an effect not seen
in our in vivo system.

Experiments dealing with the effects of DBcAMP on renin secretion have not been reported previously. The greater lipid solubility
of this compound as well as its relative resistance to breakdown by
phosphodiesterase (Posternak et al., 1962), as compared to cAMP, may
have allowed DBcAMP to accumulate in cells in sufficient quantities
to exert an effect on renin release. This could explain why an effect was seen with DBcAMP but not with cAMP. If such an assumption
is correct, our results would support a role of the adenyl cyclase
system in renin release. DBcAMP has been shown to mimic the effects
of catecholamines in some systems where catecholamine effects are
mediated by formation of intracellular cAMP (Henion et al., 1967).

From the data in Table III it is apparent that DBcAMP is not
affecting renin secretion through changes in systemic blood pressure
or plasma sodium concentration. The renin changes are, however,
accompanied by significant decreases in plasma potassium concentration. Although no studies have been reported associating acute
hypokalemia with increased PRA, Abbrecht and Vander (1970) have
reported an increase in PRA in dogs within 2 days of chronic potassium deprivation. On the other hand, a similar decrease of plasma
potassium concentration was observed during 5'-AMP infusion (Table
I) but in this case was associated with a decrease in PRA.

Theophylline was not thought to be responsible for the renin
rise seen with DBcAMP since theophylline was also administered with
the other two nucleotides at times when no changes in PRA were seen.
However, DBcAMP was always the last nucleotide administered and the
effect of theophylline on renin has been reported to continue for
some time after the infusion is stopped (see Reid et al., this volume). Therefore, it was thought possible that the effects on PRA

of DBcAMP were actually a delayed response to the three separate infusions of theophylline. For this reason the experiments in Section B were performed. In agreement with Reid et al. (this volume) and Winer et al. (1969b), our results indicate that the administration of theophylline can cause a significant increase in PRA without a concomitant decrease in blood pressure or plasma sodium or potassium concentration. Of importance also though, is the fact that the PRA level at the 60 minute time period in Table IV (30 minutes after the third infusion of theophylline was stopped) was not significantly elevated above its 0 time value. From this we conclude that the rise in PRA at this time period after DBcAMP infusion was due to some action of the nucleotide itself.

Our final series of experiments (Section C) indicated that the intrarenal administration of DBcAMP plus theophylline was accompanied by marked changes in urinary excretion of sodium, potassium and water. These changes could argue against a direct effect of DBcAMP on renin release or simply be simultaneous but unrelated effects of the nucleotide. Hypovolemia has been suggested to be a stimulus to renin secretion (Vander, 1967) and the urine volume in our dogs, already volume depleted after 1 week of a low-sodium diet, would indicate further volume depletion. In general, increased PRA has been associated with decreased urinary sodium excretion as opposed to the elevations seen in our experiments (see Vander, 1967). However, the presence of the diuretic, theophylline, might have blocked sodium reabsorption by the macula densa cells. Thus the effect of DBcAMP plus theophylline on renin in our experiments could be explained according to the macula densa theory as most recently defined by Vander (1967). It is of interest that the results of the function studies reported here are in good agreement with those recently published by Gill and Casper (1971) except for the urinary electrolyte changes. This difference might be explained by the presence of theophylline in our experiments.

SUMMARY

The cyclic nucleotide DBcAMP at a dose of 2.5 mg/min can increase PRA when administered with theophylline into the renal artery of uninephrectomized, sodium deplete dogs. This effect occurs slowly and is accompanied by a significant decrease in plasma potassium concentration as well as marked increases in urinary excretion of sodium, potassium and water. Thus it is not possible to state that DBcAMP acts directly on renin secreting cells; the increased PRA may have been due to some indirect effect of the nucleotide on, for example, electrolyte excretion. Equimolar doses of 5'-AMP and cAMP had no effect on PRA inspite of a significant decrease in plasma potassium concentration with the 2.5 mg dose of 5'-AMP. Theophylline administration alone also increased PRA but this effect was not thought to account for the rise in PRA during DBcAMP infusion.

ACKNOWLEDGEMENTS

This research was supported by USPHS Grants AM13548 and GM
0322.   The generous gift of Lonalac by Dr. John B. Mitchell of Mead
Johnson Research Labs is gratefully acknowledged.   In addition, we
are grateful for the expert technical assistance of Miss V.M.
Brorsson and Miss Jane Jackson.

REFERENCES

Abbrecht, P.H. and Vander, A.J.(1970).Effects of chronic potassium
    deficiency on plasma renin activity. J. Clin. Invest. 49: 1510-
    1516.
Allison, D.J., Clayton, P.L., Passo, S.S. and Assaykeen, T.A.(1970).
    The effect of isoproterenol and adrenergic blocking agents on
    plasma renin activity and renal function in anesthetized dogs.
    Fed. Proc. 29:782 (Abstract).
Assaykeen, T.A., Otsuka, K. and Ganong, W.F.(1968). Rate of disap-
    pearance of exogenous dog renin from the plasma of nephrectomized
    dogs. Proc. Soc. Exptl. Biol. Med. 127:306-310.
Boucher, R., Veyrat, R., deChamplain, J. and Genest, J.(1964). New
    procedures for measurement of human plasma angiotensin and renin
    activity levels. Can. Med. Assoc. J. 90:194-201.
Butcher, R.W. and Sutherland, E.W.(1962). Adenosine 3',5'-monophos-
    phate in biological materials. I. Purification and properties of
    cyclic 3',5'-nucleotide phosphodiesterase and use of this enzyme
    to characterize adenosine 3',5'-phosphate in human urine. J.
    Biol. Chem.237:1244-1250.
Fjeldbo, W. and Stamey, T.A.(1968). Adapted method for determination
    of inulin in serum and urine with an AutoAnalyzer. J. Lab. Clin.
    Med. 72:353-358.
Gill, J.R. and Casper, A.G.T.(1971). Renal effects of adenosine 3',
    5'-cyclic monophosphate and dibutyryl adenosine 3',5'-cyclic
    monophosphate. J. Clin. Invest.50:1231-1240.
Goldstein, A.(1964). Biostatistics. The MacMillan Co., New York.
Harvey, R.B. and Brothers, A.J. (1962). Renal extraction of para-
    aminohippurate and creatinine measured by continuous in vivo
    sampling of arterial and renal-vein blood. Ann. N.Y. Acad. Sci.
    102:46-54.
Henion, W.F., Sutherland, E.W. and Posternak, Th. (1967). Effects of
    derivatives of adenosine 3',5'-phosphate on liver slices and in-
    tact animals. Biochim. Biophys. Acta 148:106-113.
Higashi, A. and Peters, F.(1950). A rapid colorimetric method for
    determination of inulin in plasma and urine. J. Lab. Clin. Med.
    35:475-482.
Michelakis, A.M., Caudle, J. and Liddle, G.W.(1969). In vitro stim-
    ulation of renin production by epinephrine, norepinephrine and
    cyclic AMP. Proc. Soc. Exptl. Biol. Med. 130:748-753.

Posternak, Th., Sutherland, E.W. and Henion, W.F. (1962). Deriva-
    tives of cyclic 3',5'-adenosine monophosphate. Biochim. Biophys.
    Acta 65:558-560.
Reid, I.A. and Ganong, W.F.(1971). Effect of theophylline on renin
    secretion. Fed. Proc. 30:449 (Abstract).
Robison, G.A., Butcher, R.W. and Sutherland, E.W.(1967). Adenyl
    cyclase as an adrenergic receptor. Ann. N.Y. Acad. Sci. 139:703-
    723.
Robison, G.A., Butcher, R.W. and Sutherland, E.W.(1968). Cyclic
    AMP. Ann. Rev. Biochem. 37:149-174.
Stockigt, J.R., Collins, R.D. and Biglieri, E.G.(1971). Determina-
    tion of plasma renin concentration by angiotensin I immunoassay.
    Circulation Res. 28&29(Suppl. II):175-189.
Tagawa, H. and Vander, A.J.(1970). Effects of adenosine compounds
    on renal function and renin secretion in dogs. Circulation Res.
    26:327-338.
Vander, A.J.(1967). Control of renin release. Physiol. Rev. 47:
    359-382.
Winer, A.J., Burch, B.H., Chokshi, D.S. and Freedman, A.D.(1969a).
    Cyclic AMP stimulation of renin secretion. Program of the 51st
    Meeting of the Endocrine Society, New York, N.Y., p.100(Abstract)
Winer, N., Chokshi, D.S., Yoon, M.S. and Freedman, A.D.(1969b).
    Adrenergic receptor mediation of renin secretion. J. Clin.
    Endocrinol. Metab. 29:1168-1175.

EFFECT OF BETA-ADRENERGIC STIMULATION ON RENIN RELEASE

I.A. Reid, R.W. Schrier and L.E. Earley

Departments of Physiology and Medicine and the

Cardiovascular Research Institute, University of

California, San Francisco, California

INTRODUCTION

There are now several lines of evidence which suggest that the sympathetic nervous system plays a role in the regulation of renin secretion, and that two pathways, namely the renal sympathetic nerves and circulating catecholamines, are involved (Assaykeen and Ganong, 1971). Recently, considerable attention has been focused on the mechanism by which the renal nerves and circulating catecholamines may increase the secretion of renin. Although it appears likely that the sympathetic nervous system indirectly affects the secretion of renin through changes in renal hemodynamics and sodium excretion (Vander, 1965), there is also some evidence that renin secretion may increase in the absence of changes in renal function (Bunag et al., 1966; Ueda et al., 1968; Johnson et al., 1971; Martin and White, 1971).

There is also some evidence concerning the nature of the adrenergic receptor involved in the renin response to sympathetic stimulation. A number of stimuli which increase the release of renin may be inhibited by β-adrenergic blocking drugs, but not α-blocking drugs, suggesting that a β-adrenergic receptor is involved (Alexandre et al., 1970; Assaykeen et al., 1970; Passo et al., 1971) In general, experiments in which the effects of catecholamines on renin secretion have been studied support the β-receptor concept, although many of these experiments have been complicated by changes in blood pressure and renal function and are therefore often difficult to interpret in terms of the specific pathway involved.

49

Also of considerable interest is the location of this postulated β-receptor. The juxtaglomerular cells appear to be sympathetically innervated (Wagermark et al., 1968) and since certain sympathetic stimuli may increase renin secretion without significantly altering renal function, it has been suggested that the β-receptor is located within the juxtaglomerular apparatus (Assaykeen and Ganong, 1971). Experiments involving either intravenous or intrarenal infusion of catecholamines have neither proven nor disproven this hypothesis because of the changes in systemic and renal hemodynamics which usually accompany the infusion. For example it has been reported that infusion of isoproterenol directly into the renal artery does increase renin release (Ayers et al., 1969; Allison et al., 1970), but these experiments were performed with doses of the drug which are known to produce falls in blood pressure, plasma potassium concentration or urinary sodium excretion, each of which may stimulate the release of renin (Vander, 1967; Brunner et al., 1970). With the aim of obtaining more information concerning the nature and the location of the adrenergic receptor which may be involved in the control of renin secretion, we have performed two series of experiments. In the first series, the effect of theophylline on renin secretion was investigated. In some tissues, this drug mimics the effect of β-adrenergic stimulation to increase intracellular cyclic AMP by inhibiting phosphodiesterase (Butcher and Sutherland, 1962). Therefore, if a β-receptor is involved in renin release, and if this effect is mediated by cyclic AMP, it might be expected that theophylline administration would stimulate renin release. An abstract reporting the results of the theophylline study has been published (Reid and Ganong, 1971). A second series of experiments was undertaken with isoproterenol to examine whether β-adrenergic stimulation can increase renin secretion in the absence of changes in renal perfusion pressure and renal hemodynamics. A second purpose of these experiments was to determine if this β-adrenergic effect occurs directly within the kidney, or results from some extrarenal effect of β-adrenergic stimulation. This was done by comparing the effect on renin release of intravenous infusion and renal arterial infusion of isoproterenol. The intrarenal doses were such that systemic effects of β-adrenergic stimulation were avoided and yet the intrarenal concentration of the drug was in excess of that achieved during the intravenous infusion. To examine the importance of the renal innervation, experiments were also performed in animals in which one or both kidneys were denervated. Since β-adrenergic stimulation is associated with antidiuresis, studies were also performed in animals in which the hypophyseal-hypothalamic neural pathways were abolished so that any interaction between ADH and renin secretion could be excluded.

METHODS

Theophylline

These experiments were performed in six male dogs anesthetized with pentobarbital. After two control arterial blood samples were collected, theophylline ethylenediamine (Aminophyllin, Searle) was infused intravenously in a dose of 7 mg/kg over 15 minutes. Six additional blood samples were then collected during the following two hours. This protocol was also performed in seven dogs receiving propranolol (0.6 mg/kg followed by infusion at 0.3 mg/kg/hr) as well as in seven dogs treated with phenoxybenzamine (2.5 mg/kg administered in a single dose). Arterial blood pressure was recorded throughout the experiment but renal function studies were not performed. All blood samples were analyzed for plasma renin activity using a radioimmunoassay for angiotensin I (Stockigt et al., 1971). Plasma epinephrine and norepinephrine were measured by a modification of the ethylenediamine method (Goldfien et al., 1961). Plasma sodium and potassium concentration were measured by flame photometry.

Isoproterenol

Thirteen dogs were used in this series of experiments. In eight, one or both kidneys were denervated and in six the hypothalamus and pituitary were removed prior to the experiment. Catheters were placed in both ureters and renal veins to permit bilateral renal function studies. In the animals in which isoproterenol was infused intravenously, a clamp was placed around the aorta above the renal arteries in order to allow control of renal perfusion pressure. Blood pressure was recorded continuously from a brachial artery and from the aorta below the clamp. Water diuresis was induced by administration of 2.5% dextrose in water. Urine was collected at 10 min intervals throughout the experiment and arterial and renal venous blood samples were collected at the mid-point of alternate periods. Cardiac output was measured during alternate periods using the dye-dilution technique. Arterial and renal venous blood samples for renin assay were collected during the control period, 20-50 min after starting the infusion and 20-60 min after stopping the infusion.

In five experiments, isoproterenol was infused directly into the left renal artery in doses ranging from 0.009 - 0.036 µg/kg/min. In one of these experiments, phenoxybenzamine was infused into the left renal artery in a dose of 0.09 µg/kg/min throughout the experiment. In 14 experiments, isoproterenol was infused into a femoral vein in doses ranging from 0.009 - 0.036 µg/kg/min, except in two experiments in which doses of 0.072 and 0.144 µg/kg/min were used. In order to avoid a fall in renal perfusion pressure during the infusion, the renal perfusion pressure was lowered 15-20 mm Hg below systemic pressure before the control period and maintained at this value throughout the experiment by appropriate adjustment of the aortic clamp.

Plasma and urine samples were analyzed for inulin, para-aminohippuric acid (PAH), osmolality, sodium and potassium, and hematocrit and plasma protein concentration were measured. Plasma renin activity was measured by immunoassay and a rate of renin secretion was calculated from the renal arteriovenous difference in plasma renin activity and renal plasma flow, and expressed as PRA units (ng/ml/3hr)/min.

All results are expressed as the mean ± the standard error (S.E.) of the mean. Statistical analysis between groups of animals was performed using the t-test. The paired t-test was used for comparisons within groups.

RESULTS

Theophylline

The effect of the theophylline on plasma renin activity, plasma epinephrine and blood pressure in six anesthetized dogs, is shown in Figure 1.

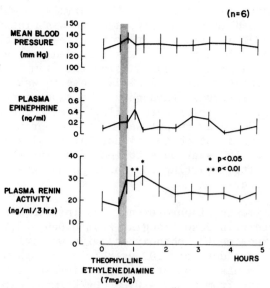

Figure 1.   The effect of theophylline infusion on plasma renin activity, plasma epinephrine concentration and mean blood pressure.

Plasma renin activity increased from 17.4 ± 3.8 (S.E.) to 29.1 ± 6.3 ng/ml/3hr during the theophylline infusion and was significantly higher than the control values 30 and 45 min after the start of the infusion. There were no significant changes in blood pressure or plasma epinephrine concentration during the experiment. Plasma norepinephrine, sodium and potassium concentrations were also unchanged.

Theophylline and Propranolol. These results are summarized in Figure 2. In the propranolol-treated dogs, the plasma renin activity before theophylline was approximately one half the values in untreated dogs, although this difference was not statistically significant. Theophylline infusion was associated with a significant increase in plasma renin activity, in the absence of changes in plasma epinephrine concentration or blood pressure. There were also no changes in plasma norepinephrine, sodium or potassium concentration.

Theophylline and Phenoxybenzamine. In the dogs treated with phenoxybenzamine, mean blood pressure was lower and plasma epinephrine was higher than in the untreated dogs, while the control plasma renin activity was similar in both groups (Figure 3). Theophylline infusion caused no further significant changes in plasma epinephrine concentration or blood pressure, but increased renin activity more than two-fold. In the phenoxybenzamine-treated dogs there were no significant changes in plasma norepinephrine, sodium or potassium concentration.

Isoproterenol

The effects of intravenous and intrarenal isoproterenol infusion on arterial plasma renin activity are shown in Figure 4. In all animals, intravenous infusion produced reversible increases in plasma renin activity - the mean value for the group as a whole rose from 14.2 ± 2.8 (S.E.) to 39.3 ± 5.9 ng/ml/3hr (P< 0.001) during the infusion and decreased to 20.8 ± 3.5 ng/ml/3hr following completion of the infusion (P< 0.001). In contrast, there were no significant changes in plasma renin activity following intrarenal infusion - the mean values before, during and after the infusion were 19.8 ± 10.5, 22.6 ± 9.4, and 22.0 ± 9.0 ng/ml/3hr respectively. These values include the animal which received intrarenal phenoxybenzamine throughout the experiment.

Figure 5 shows the effects of intravenous and intrarenal isoproterenol infusion on renin secretion rate. Intravenous infusion produced reversible increases in renin secretion rate in 24 of 28 kidneys - the mean value rose from 1413 ± 298 to 5445 ± 1158 units/min during the infusion (P< 0.001) and decreased to 1590 ± 265 units/min when the infusion was stopped (P< 0.005). The magnitude of the increase in secretion rate in the denervated kidneys was almost identical to that in the intact kidneys. In the innervated

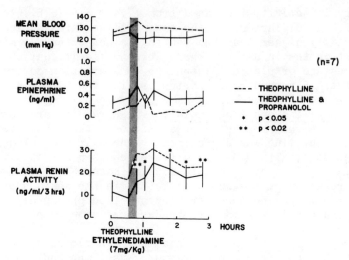

Figure 2. The effect of theophylline infusion on plasma renin
           activity, plasma epinephrine concentration and mean
           blood pressure in dogs treated with propranolol. The
           responses in the dogs that were not treated with
           propranolol are also shown for comparison.

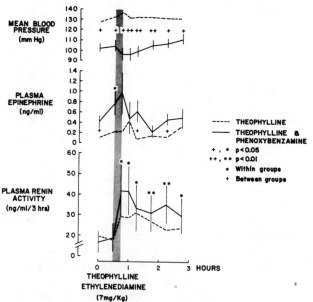

Figure 3. The effect of theophylline infusion on plasma renin
           activity, plasma epinephrine concentration and mean
           blood pressure in dogs treated with phenoxybenzamine.
           The responses in the dogs that were not treated with
           phenoxybenzamine are also shown for comparison.

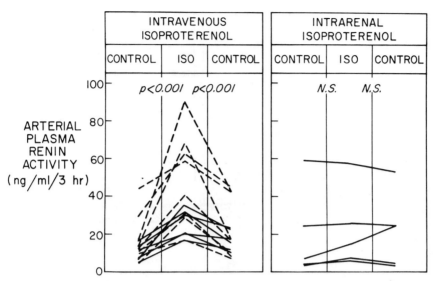

Figure 4. Comparison of the effects of intravenous and intrarenal
           isoproterenol infusion on plasma renin activity. In
           the intravenous infusion experiments, the broken lines
           indicate the animals from which the pituitary and hypo-
           thalamus had been removed and the unbroken lines
           indicate intact animals.

kidneys, the secretion rate increased from 1753 ± 409 to 6485 ± 1780
units/min during the infusion (P< 0.02) and decreased to 2025 ± 402
after the infusion (P< 0.05). The corresponding values for the
denervated kidneys were 1159 ± 422, 4665 ± 1545 (P< 0.02) and
1264 ± 339 (P< 0.05). In contrast, intrarenal infusion produced no
consistent changes in renin secretion rate, either in the infused
kidneys, or in the contralateral kidneys. The mean secretion rates
in the infused kidneys before, during and after the infusion were
1020 ± 729, 2257 ± 654 and 2012 ± 645 units/min respectively, and
in the contralateral kidneys were 1916 ± 888, 2034 ± 679 and
2419 ± 948 units/min. None of these changes was statistically
significant.

    In Figure 6, the effects of intravenous and intrarenal iso-
proterenol infusion on cardiac output and arterial pressure are
compared. Intravenous infusion produced a significant, reversible
increase in cardiac output and a slight, but statistically significant decrease in systemic pressure. Renal perfusion pressure was
maintained at a constant level throughout the experiment. Intrarenal isoproterenol caused no significant changes in cardiac output
or arterial pressure.

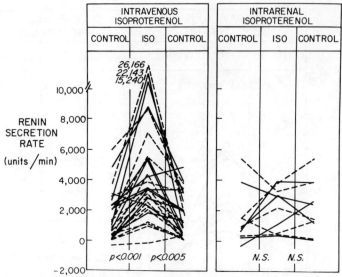

Figure 5. Comparison of the effects of intravenous and intrarenal isoproterenol infusion on renin secretion rate. In the intravenous infusion experiments, the broken lines indicate denervated kidneys and the unbroken lines indicate intact kidneys. In the intrarenal infusion experiments, the unbroken lines indicate the infused kidneys, and the broken lines indicate the contralateral kidney.

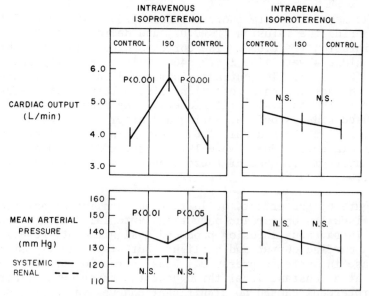

Figure 6. Comparison of the effects of intravenous and intrarenal isoproterenol infusion on cardiac output and mean arterial pressure.

The renal hemodynamic changes following isoproterenol infusion are summarized in Figure 7. Intravenous infusion produced no significant change in renal plasma flow, but caused slight increases in GFR and filtration fraction which remained elevated after the infusion was stopped. A significant increase in renal vascular resistance occurred following cessation of the infusion. None of these parameters showed any significant changes during, or after intrarenal infusion of the drug in either the infused or contralateral kidneys.

In Figure 8, the changes in urinary solute and water excretion are summarized. During intravenous infusion, there were no significant changes in sodium or potassium excretion, but after the infusion the excretion of both these ions increased. Intrarenal infusion was associated with small increases in sodium excretion in both the infused and contralateral kidneys, but these increases persisted after stopping the infusion. There were no consistent changes in potassium excretion during the intrarenal infusion. Intravenous infusion produced a decrease in free-water clearance which was proportional to an increase in urine osmolality suggesting a release of ADH. In animals from which the pituitary and hypothalamus had been removed intravenous isoproterenol had no effect on free-water clearance. Infusion of isoproterenol into the renal artery had no effect on free-water clearance or urine osmolality in either the infused or contralateral kidneys.

Changes in blood composition are summarized in Figure 9. Intravenous infusion produced a small, reversible increase in hematocrit which did not occur during the intrarenal infusion. Plasma protein concentration tended to progressively decrease during both the intravenous and intrarenal infusion experiments: plasma sodium also tended to decrease progressively in both groups of experiments, but this change was statistically significant only in the intravenous experiments. There were no significant changes in plasma potassium concentration in either series of experiments.

DISCUSSION

The demonstration in the present study that the intravenous infusion of theophylline significantly increases plasma renin activity is compatible with the hypothesis that the intracellular concentration of 3' 5' adenosine monophosphate (cyclic AMP) may act as a mediator of renin release. This interpretation is based on the known effect of theophylline to inhibit in some tissues the degradation of cyclic AMP by phosphodiesterase (Butcher and Sutherland, 1962). The suggestion that this may be the pathway by which theophylline stimulated a release of renin accrues from the observations that no changes occurred in the several well-known variables that effect the release of renin. Arterial pressure and plasma potassium

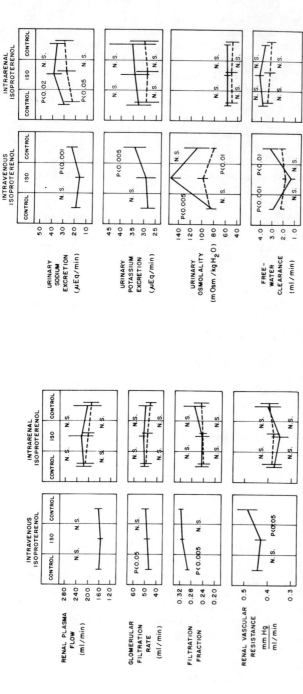

Figure 7.   Comparison of the effects of intravenous and intrarenal isoproterenol
infusion on renal hemodynamics. In
the intrarenal infusion experiments,
the unbroken lines indicate the
infused kidneys and the broken lines
indicate the contralateral kidney.

Figure 8.   Comparison of the effects of intravenous and intrarenal isoproterenol infusion on urinary solute and water excretion. In the intravenous infusion experiments, the broken lines indicate
the animals from which the pituitary
and hypothalamus had been removed and
the unbroken lines indicate intact
animals. In the intrarenal infusion
experiments, the unbroken lines indicate the infused kidneys and the broken
lines indicate the contralateral kidneys.

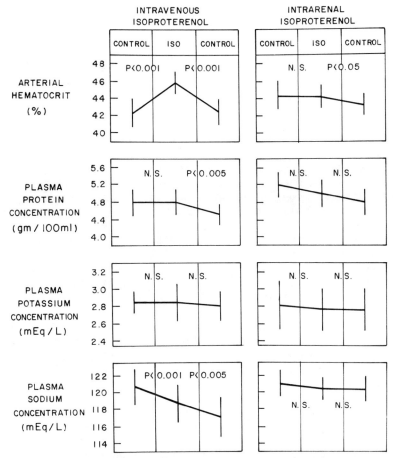

Figure 9.   Comparison of the effects of intravenous and
intrarenal isoproterenol infusion on blood
composition.

concentration did not decrease and there was no consistent increase
in plasma concentrations of epinephrine or norepinephrine. Moreover,
the effect of theophylline on plasma renin activity was not affected
by either alpha- or beta-adrenergic blocking agents. Since beta-
adrenergic stimulation has been shown to increase adenyl cyclase
activity and cyclic AMP production, some authors have suggested that
adenyl cyclase is a beta-adrenergic receptor, and cyclic AMP is the
intracellular messenger (Robison and Sutherland, 1970). Although
beta-adrenergic blockade would be expected to inhibit the effect of
beta-receptor mediated stimulation of cyclic AMP production, the
effect of theophylline to increase cyclic AMP may not be blocked
since its effect is by inhibiting the breakdown of cyclic AMP by

phosphodiesterase. Since this effect of theophylline occurs independently of activation of adenyl cyclase it should not be affected by beta-adrenergic blocking agents.

Although renal hemodynamics were not measured in the experiments with theophylline it does not seem likely that a decrease in delivery of sodium to the macula densa was the stimulus for the release of renin during theophylline infusion. Theophylline has been shown to increase glomerular filtration rate (Kleeman et al., 1958) and decrease proximal sodium reabsorption (Stribrna et al., 1968) both of which would be expected to increase the delivery of sodium to the macula densa during theophylline infusion. Therefore, by elimination of the recognized stimuli for renin release the present results are consistent with the view that the effect of theophylline to stimulate a release of renin may relate to an effect of the agent to increase cyclic AMP either in the cells of the juxtaglomerular apparatus or at some extrarenal site which secondarily leads to a release of renin. Alternatively, the effects of theophylline on the release of renin could be due to some less specific and undefined effect of the drug. Additional studies will be necessary to further delineate the mechanisms involved.

The results of the experiments with intravenous and intrarenal infusion of isoproterenol demonstrated that extrarenal mechanisms are involved in the effect of beta-adrenergic stimulation to increase the secretion of renin. Moreover, the effect of intravenous isoproterenol to increase renin secretion was not associated with decreases in renal perfusion pressure or plasma potassium concentration. Although previous studies suggest that isoproterenol infusion may cause a decrease in plasma potassium concentration (Todd and Vick, 1971) which could constitute a stimulus to renin release (Brunner et al., 1970), the smaller doses of the drug used in the present study were not associated with changes in plasma potassium concentration. Since the effect of intravenous isoproterenol to decrease total peripheral resistance was generally greater than the drug's effect to increase cardiac output, a small fall in mean arterial pressure usually occurred. However, an effect of the agent on renal perfusion pressure was avoided by appropriately adjusting the suprarenal clamp. Nevertheless, the possibility exists that the fall in systemic blood pressure and/or the increased cardiac output were important in initiating an extrarenal mechanism leading to the stimulation of renin secretion. Support for this possibility was found in the results obtained during the intrarenal infusion of isoproterenol. Despite the intrarenal infusion of isoproterenol in amounts comparable to those infused intravenously, the intrarenal infusions did not affect systemic hemodynamics or the secretion of renin. This lack of systemic effects of isoproterenol during renal arterial infusion suggests that the kidney is very efficient in either inactivating or removing isoproterenol from blood. To what extent tissue uptake, metabolism and excretion are involved in this process is currently under investigation in our laboratory.

The present results also emphasize the importance of measuring cardiac output in order to adequately evaluate systemic effects of the drug. In some studies involving intravenous infusion, the effect of isoproterenol to increase cardiac output was inversely proportional to the decreased total peripheral resistance with the result that arterial pressure was unchanged. In the absence of measurements of cardiac output it would appear in such experiments that the intravenous infusion of isoproterenol had no effect on systemic hemodynamics and, therefore, no hemodynamic differences between the two routes of infusion would have been observed.

In addition to the different effects of intrarenal and intravenous infusion of isoproterenol on systemic hemodynamics, other differences were also noted which could be involved in the extrarenal pathway of beta-adrenergic stimulation to increase renin secretion. Small increases in hematocrit occurred during intravenous, but not intrarenal, infusion of isoproterenol. However, it seems unlikely that these small changes in hematocrit could account for the large increase in renin release. Also, intravenous, but not intrarenal, infusion of isoproterenol was associated with an antidiuresis resembling an effect of ADH. This effect was abolished by removing the sources of production and release of ADH in the pituitary and hypothalamus supporting the conclusion that the antidiuresis was mediated by ADH. Thus, increased circulatory levels of ADH could have influenced the release of renin in some of the experiments involving the intravenous infusion of isoproterenol. However, this possibility was excluded in other experiments since in the animals in which the hypophyseal-hypothalamic neural system had been abolished the effect on the release of renin still occurred and even appeared to be somewhat accentuated (Figure 4). A possible explanation for this apparent accentuation of the release of renin is found in the previous evidence that ADH may depress plasma renin activity (Tagawa et al., 1971). Thus, ADH release in the intact animals may have blunted the effect of intravenous isoproterenol to increase the release of renin.

At the doses used in the present experiments neither intravenous nor intrarenal isoproterenol significantly altered renal hemodynamics. Furthermore, the effect of intravenous isoproterenol to stimulate the release of renin was not dependent on renal innervation. However, intravenous isoproterenol always decreased total peripheral resistance and sometimes decreased arterial pressure, changes which could result in an increased adrenal secretion of epinephrine, and to a lesser degree norepinephrine. Thus, increased circulating catecholamines may have been involved in stimulating the increased release of renin. However, if the same pathway mediates the effect of isoproterenol and theophylline to increase the release of renin, some factor(s) other than circulating catecholamines would seem to be involved, since in the experiments with theophylline measured increases in catecholamines were not consistently associated with the increase in plasma renin activity. Another possibility that cannot be dismissed is that some other, as yet unidentified, circulating renin-stimulating substance is involved in the effect of beta-adrenergic stimulation to increase the release of renin. Such a humoral effect of intravenous isoproterenol on the release of renin could be initiated by the alterations in systemic hemodynamics. Lastly, it is tempting to postulate that this extrarenal reflex stimulation of renin release involves the accumulation of cyclic AMP, probably within the cardiovascular system, which in the case of isoproterenol results from beta-adrenergic activation of adenyl cyclase and in the case of theophylline from the inhibition of phosphodiesterase. We are presently investigating the possibility that theophylline produces changes in cardiac output and peripheral resistance which are qualitatively similar to those observed during the intravenous infusion of isoproterenol. This will be a first and necessary step in establishing that the two agents lead to increased release of renin through a common extrarenal pathway.

ACKNOWLEDGEMENTS

The work reported was supported by USPHS Grants AM06704, AM12753 and HE13319-01A1, Grant NGR05025007 from the National Aeronautics and Space Administration and the L.J. and Mary C. Skaggs Foundation. Dr. Reid is a Bay Area Heart Research Committee Fellow. Dr. Schrier is an established Investigator of the American Heart Association.

The authors would like to express their appreciation for excellent technical assistance from Judith H. Harbottle and Lisbeth Streiff.

REFERENCES

Alexandre, J.M., J. Menard, C. Chevillard and H. Schmitt (1970) Increased plasma renin activity induced in rats by physostigmine and effects of alpha- and beta-blocking drugs thereon. European J. Pharmacol. 12, 127.

Allison, D.J., P.L. Clayton, S.S. Passo and T.A. Assaykeen (1970). The effect of isoproterenol and adrenergic blocking agents on plasma renin activity and renal function in anesthetized dogs. Fed. Proc. 29, 782 (Abstract).

Assaykeen, T.A., P.L. Clayton, A. Goldfien and W.F. Ganong (1970). Effect of alpha- and beta-adrenergic blocking agents on the renin response to hypoglycemia and epinephrine in dogs. Endocrinology 87, 1318.

Assaykeen, T.A. and W.F. Ganong (1971). The sympathetic nervous
    system and renin secretion, in: Frontiers in Neuroendocrinology,
    eds. L. Martini and W.F. Ganong, (Oxford University Press,
    New York) pp. 67-102.
Ayers, C.R., R.H. Harris and L.E. Lefer (1969). Control of renin
    release in experimental hypertension. Circulation Res. 24 & 25
    (Suppl. I), 103.
Brunner, H.R., L. Baer, J.E. Sealey, J.G.G. Ledingham and
    J.H. Laragh (1970). The influence of potassium administration
    and of potassium deprivation on plasma renin in normal and
    hypertensive subjects. J. Clin. Invest. 49, 2128.
Bunag, R.D., I.H. Page and J.W. McCubbin (1966). Neural stimulation
    of release of renin. Circulation Res. 19, 851.
Butcher, R.W. and E.W. Sutherland (1962). Adenosine 3', 5'-phosphate
    in biological materials. J. Biol. Chem. 237, 1244.
Goldfien, A., S. Zileli, D. Goodman and G.W. Thorn (1961). The
    estimation of epinephrine and norepinephrine in human plasma.
    J. Clin. Endocrinol. 21, 281.
Johnson, J.A., J.O. Davis and R.T. Witty (1971). Control of renin
    secretion by the renal sympathetic nerves. Physiologist 14,
    168 (Abstract).
Kleeman, C.R., M.H. Maxwell and R.E. Rockney (1958). Mechanisms of
    impaired water excretion in adrenal and pituitary insufficiency.
    1. The role of altered glomerular filtration rate and solute
    excretion. J. Clin. Invest. 37, 1799.
Martin, D.M. and F.N. White (1971). Evidence for direct neural
    release of renin. Fed. Proc. 30, 431 (Abstract).
Passo, S.S., T.A. Assaykeen, A. Goldfien and W.F. Ganong (1971).
    Effect of alpha- and beta-adrenergic blocking agents on the
    increase in renin secretion produced by stimulation of the
    medulla oblongata in dogs. Neuroendocrinology 7, 97.
Reid, I.A. and W.F. Ganong (1971). Effect of theophylline on renin
    secretion. Fed. Proc. 30, 449 (Abstract).
Robison, G.A. and E.W. Sutherland (1970). Sympathin E,,Sympathin I,
    and the intracellular level of cyclic AMP. Circulation Res.
    26 & 27 (Suppl.I), 147.
Stockigt, J.R., R.D. Collins and E.G. Biglieri (1971). Determination
    of plasma renin concentration by angiotensin I immunoassay.
    Circulation Res. 28 & 29 (Suppl. II), 175.
Stribrna, V.J., O. Schuck and I. Sotornik (1968). Veranderungen der
    tubularen Natriumresorption nach Aminophyllin und Polythiazid,
    Zschr. inn. Med., Jahrg. 23, 100.
Tagawa, H., A.J. Vander, J.P. Bonjour, and R.L. Malvin (1971).
    Inhibition of renin secretion by vasopressin in unanesthetized
    sodium-deprived dogs. Am. J. Physiol. 220, 949.
Todd, E.P. and R.L. Vick (1971). Kalemotropic effect of epinephrine:
    analysis with adrenergic agonists and antagonists. Am. J.
    Physiol. 220, 1964.

Ueda, H., Y. Hisakazu, Y. Takabatake, M. Iizuka, T. Iizuka, M. Ihori
    and Y. Sakamoto (1970). Observations on the mechanism of renin
    release by catecholamines. Circulation Res. 26 & 27 (Suppl. II),
    195.
Vander, A.J. (1967). Control of renin release. Physiol. Rev. 47,
    349.
Wagermark, J., U. Ungerstedt and A. Llungquist (1968). Sympathetic
    innervation of the juxtaglomerular cells of the kidney.
    Circulation Res. 22, 149.

EFFECTS OF ADRENERGIC ANTAGONISTS IN STATES OF INCREASED RENIN SECRETION

N. Winer, W.G. Walkenhorst, R. Helman and D. Lamy

Raymond H. Starr Hypertension Laboratory and the

Department of Medicine, Menorah Medical Center,

Kansas City, Missouri

We have previously shown that renin release provoked by upright posture and administration of various pharmacologic agents is inhibited by adrenergic receptor blocking agents (1). Likewise, administration of cyclic 3',5' adenosine monophosphate (cyclic AMP) and sympathomimetic amines, such as isoproterenol and norepinephrine, has also been shown to stimulate renin secretion, actions that likewise are blocked by adrenergic antagonists (2). These observations suggest that the adrenergic blockers may be inhibiting renin secretion at an intracellular site distal to cyclic AMP production and that this pathway may mediate many, if not all, stimuli for renin secretion. In the present study, we have assessed the effect of adrenergic blocking agents on a variety of other stimuli which are known to increase renin secretion; these include acute hemorrhage, adrenalectomy, chronic salt depletion and acute renal artery constriction.

METHODS

Acute Hemorrhage. Sprague Dawley rats weighing from 492 to 612 grams were anesthetized by intraperitoneal injection of sodium pentobarbital (50mg per kg). The carotid artery was cannulated with a polyethylene catheter, connected to a Sanborn Transducer (Model 267PC) with a Hewlett Packard recorder for monitoring blood pressure and heart rate. Seven ml of blood was withdrawn from the carotid artery over a two minute period and placed into iced heparinized tubes. The plasma was removed for determination of renin activity (PRA). Ten minutes later, blood pressure and pulse rate were again determined and a second blood sample was obtained for measurement of PRA.

Adrenalectomy. Rats weighing 125 to 150 g were anesthetized as above and bilateral adrenalectomy was performed. Within 24 hr the animals were again anesthetized, the carotid artery was cannulated for recording of blood pressure and pulse rate and blood was drawn for determination of PRA.

Chronic Salt Depletion. Rats were placed on a sodium deficient diet (Hartroft formula, Catalogue No. 17950, General Biochemicals) (3). After one week on this diet, the carotid artery was cannulated for recording of blood pressure and pulse rate and blood was obtained for determination of PRA.

Renal Artery Constriction. Mongrel dogs (15 to 20 kg) on an unrestricted dietary sodium intake, were anesthetized with sodium pentobarbital, 30mg per kg i.v. with supplements given as necessary. Through a subcostal approach, a catheter was placed in the left renal vein in order to obtain samples for determination of renal vein renin activity (RVRA) and kept open by constant infusion of normal saline at a rate approximately equal to the urine flow. In addition, a polyethylene catheter was placed into the ureter for collection and measurement of urine volume. Blood pressure was monitored by a catheter in the femoral artery. A Goldblatt clamp was placed on the renal artery and alternately opened and closed at 15 minute intervals to allow for control periods and periods of renal artery constriction. Renal blood flow was measured by standard PAH clearance methods and glomerular filtration rate was determined by the creatinine clearance. Urinary sodium excretion was measured by flame photometry and PRA was determined by the bio-assay method of Gunnells et al. (4). Renin secretion was calculated as the product of renal blood flow and the arterial PRA-RVRA renal difference.

As shown previously (2), the use of plasma containing adrenergic blocking agents had no effect on measured PRA. Statistical significance was determined by means of Student's t test.

RESULTS

Acute Hemorrhage. (Table 1 and Figure 1) Following rapid withdrawal of 7.0ml of blood, mean systemic blood pressure fell significantly from 171.1 ± 15.5 (SD) to 122.5 ± 32.5mm Hg ($p < 0.02$),while PRA rose from a mean of 270.7 ± 45.2 to 370.5 ± 27.8ng per 100ml ($p < 0.01$). Heart rate decreased from a mean of 333.5 ± 31 to 304.1 ± 51.6 beats per minute; however, the difference was not a significant one.

In rats given the α adrenergic receptor blocking agent, phentolamine, 1mg, by intraperitoneal injection 15 minutes prior to

TABLE 1

Effects of Acute Hemorrhage and Adrenergic Antagonists on Blood Pressure,
Heart Rate and Plasma Renin Activity (PRA)

	Dose (mg)*	No. of Experiments	Mean Arterial Blood Pressure (mm Hg)	Mean Heart Rate (Beats/min)	Mean PRA (ng/100 ml)
Pre-hemorrhage)	- - - - -	6	171.1 ± 15.5	333.5 ± 31.0	270.7 ± 45.2
Post-hemorrhage)			122.5 ± 32.5[b]	304.1 ± 51.6	370.5 ± 27.8[a]
Pre-hemorrhage)	phentolamine (1)	5	133.3 ± 16.8	349.8 ± 54.9	244.0 ± 5.1
Post-hemorrhage)			75.1 ± 42.0[c]	275.4 ± 53.8	267.2 ± 21.5
Pre-hemorrhage)	propranolol (0.2)	5	137.1 ± 8.9	320.2 ± 43.2	259.6 ± 15.5
Post-hemorrhage)			49.4 ± 16.7[a]	273.6 ± 44.0	267.0 ± 16.2

[a] $p < 0.01$ [b] $p < 0.02$ [c] $p < 0.05$

* Given by intraperitoneal injection 15 minutes prior to prehemorrhage measurements.
Values are mean ± SD

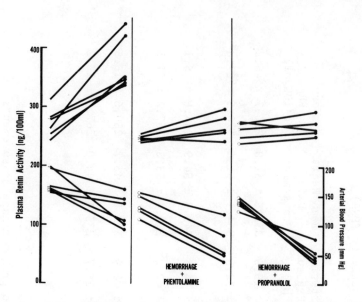

Figure 1.   The effects of acute hemorrhage and adrenergic antag-
            onists on blood pressure and plasma renin activity.
            Pre-hemorrhage values for PRA and arterial blood pres-
            sure are shown in open circles, while post-hemorrhage
            values are shown in solid circles. The intraperitoneal
            administration of phentolamine, 1mg, or propranolol,
            0.2mg, suppressed the post-hemorrhage values of plasma
            renin activity but did not prevent the fall in blood
            pressure.

cannulation of the carotid artery, mean PRA rose only slightly
following acute hemorrhage from 244.0 ± 51 to 267.2 ± 21.5 ng per
100ml ($p = 0.7$), despite a fall in mean blood pressure from $133 \pm$
16.8 to 75.1 ± 42mm Hg ($p < 0.05$). There was no significant change
in heart rate. With administration of the β adrenergic blocking
agent, propranolol, 0.2mg intraperitoneally 15 minutes before
carotid artery cannulation, mean PRA rose from 259.6 ± 15.5 to
267.0 ± 16.2ng per 100ml, while mean blood pressure fell from 137.1
± 8.9 to 49.4 ± 16.7 ($p < 0.01$). Mean heart rate did not change
significantly.

    Adrenalectomy. (Table 2 and Figure 2) Mean PRA in blood samples
obtained from rats within 24 hours of bilateral adrenalectomy was
424.7 ± 19.9ng per 100ml compared to that of intact rats in whom PRA
was 263.1 ± 15.0ng per 100ml ($p < 0.0001$). Mean arterial blood
pressure was significantly lower in adrenalectomized rats than in
the control group ($p < 0.02$).

    However, when adrenalectomized rats were given phentolamine,
1mg twice a day subcutaneously, PRA failed to rise compared to un-

TABLE 2

Effect of Adrenalectomy and Adrenergic Antagonists on
Blood Pressure, Heart Rate and Plasma Renin Activity (PRA)

	Agent (mg)*	No. of Experiments	Mean Arterial Blood Pressure (mm Hg)	Mean Heart Rate (Beats/min)	Mean PRA (ng/100 ml)
Control	-----	7	140.9 ± 34.4	426.9 ± 63.1	263.1 ± 15.0
Adrenalectomized	-----	11	102.2 ± 22.2[a]	392.2 ± 56.2	424.7 ± 19.9[c]
Adrenalectomized	phentolamine (2.0)	6	132.5 ± 25.1	366.0 ± 40.9	242.5 ± 13.1[b]
Adrenalectomized	propranolol (0.4)	8	100.0 ± 10.8[a]	385.7 ± 24.8	250.6 ± 26.9[b]

Values are means ± SD.
[a] p < 0.02 adrenalectomized rats compared to control
[b] p < 0.001 compared to adrenalectomized rats
[c] p < 0.0001 compared to control

* given subcutaneously in 2 divided doses daily.

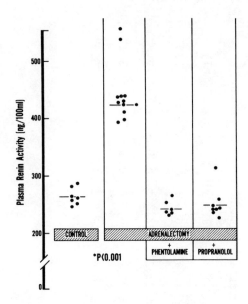

Figure 2.   The effects of adrenalectomy and adrenergic antogonists
            on plasma renin activity. Adrenalectomized rats had
            sigificantly higher plasma renin activity than intact
            rats. When adrenalectomized rats were given phentol-
            amine, 2mg daily, or propranolol, 0.4mg daily, PRA
            was suppressed to control levels.

treated adrenalectomized rats (p < 0.001). Likewise, in adrenalectomized rats given propranolol, 0.2mg twice daily, mean PRA was
250.6 ± 26.9, a significantly lower value than that of adrenalectomized rats not receiving an adrenergic blocker. Mean arterial
blood pressure in adrenalectomized propranolol-treated rats was
significantly lower than that of the control group (p < 0.02).

    Chronic Salt Depletion. (Table 3 and Figure 3) Rats fed a
sodium deficient diet for one week showed a mean PRA of 364.0 ±
25.5ng per 100ml, a significantly higher value than rats receiving
a standard Purina rat chow diet (p < 0.001). Rats receiving a low
salt diet who were given either phentolamine, 0.5mg twice daily, or
propranolol, 0.1mg twice daily, failed to show any suppression of
PRA, their mean PRA values of 405.7 ± 46.9 and 399.0 ± 29.7mg per
100ml being significantly higher than that of the Purina chow-fed
group (p < 0.001). However, when rats fed a salt deficient diet were
treated with either phentolamine, 1mg twice daily or propranolol,
0.2mg twice daily, mean PRA was suppressed to levels below that of
the control group. Mean heart rates were significantly decreased
in both the low and high dose propranolol-treated sodium deficient
rats compared to untreated rats receiving the low salt diet (p < 0.02).
No significant alterations in mean blood pressures occurred.

TABLE 3

Effect of Sodium Deficient Diet and Adrenergic Antagonists on
Blood Pressure, Heart Rate and Plasma Renin Activity (PRA)

Diet	Agent* (mg)	No. of Experiments	Mean Arterial Blood Pressure (mm Hg)	Mean Heart Rate (Beats/min)	Mean PRA (ng/100ml)
Normal	-----	7	140.9 ± 34.4	478.3 ± 29.7	263.1 ± 15.0
Low Salt	-----	7	151.0 ± 18.8	426.9 ± 63.1	364.0 ± 25.5[a]
Low Salt	phentolamine (1)	6	156.3 ± 19.2	416.0 ± 62.9	405.7 ± 46.9[a]
Low Salt	propranolol (0.2)	5	137.2 ± 9.9	370.8 ± 60.4[b]	399.0 ± 29.7[a]
Low Salt	phentolamine (2)	5	123.0 ± 35.9	467.6 ± 26.2	249.4 ± 15.5
Low Salt	propranolol (0.4)	5	115.8 ± 29.5	355.0 ± 83.7[b]	264.4 ± 46.4

Values are means ± SD.
[a] $p < 0.001$ compared to control.
[b] $p < 0.02$ compared to low salt diet.
* given subcutaneously in 2 divided doses daily.

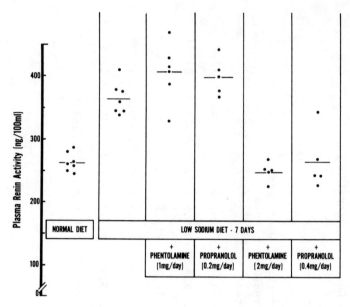

Figure 3.   The effect of sodium deficient diet and adrenergic
            antagonists on plasma renin activity. Rats subjected
            to low sodium diet for 7 days had significantly higher
            plasma renin activity than control rats. Phentolamine
            and propranolol, in the higher doses, suppressed PRA
            to the normal range.

    Renal Artery Constriction.   (Table 4, Figures 4 and 5)   In dogs
in whom renal artery constriction was produced by tightening a
Goldblatt clamp mean RVRA rose significantly from a control value
of 266.7 ± 31.5 to 435.0 ± 71.7ng per 100ml (p < 0.001). Simultaneously arterial PRA rose from 267.4 ± 28.1 to 314.4 ± 58.1ng per
100ml and then fell during the recovery period to 274.0 ± 39.3ng
per 100ml. These differences, however, were not significant.
During renal artery clamping mean renal blood flow fell from 174.1 ±
66.5 to 98.6 ± 62.7ml per min and after release of the clamp, rose
to 148.0 ± 79.1ml per min. Mean renin secretion, calculated as the
product of the renal blood flow and the arterial PRA-RVRA difference,
increased from 17.1 ± 13.8 to 138.2 ± 128.6ng per min during renal
artery constriction (p < 0.05) and declined to 22.4 ± 11.6ng per min
during the recovery period (p < 0.05). In addition, glomerular filtration rate, urine flow and urinary sodium excretion also fell significantly during the period of renal artery constriction and returned to control levels following release of the clamp. No significant
differences were observed in mean heart rate or mean arterial blood
pressure.

    When phentolamine, 8.8μg per kg per minute was infused via
the femoral vein during renal artery constriction, there were no

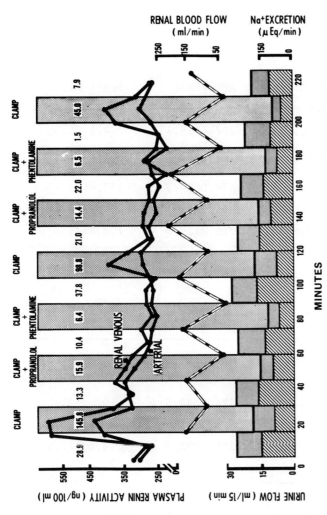

MINUTES

Figure 4. Typical experiment showing the effect of renal artery clamping on renin secretion, renal vein renin activity, arterial plasma renin activity, renal blood flow, urine flow and sodium excretion. The stippled bars represent 15 minute periods during which Goldblatt clamp was tightened; the numbers at the top represent calculated values for renin secretion; solid bars depict urine flow; cross-hatched bars represent sodium excretion. Renin secretion, RVRA and arterial PRA rose during periods of renal artery constriction, except when propranolol or phentolamine was infused. Renal blood flow, urinary flow and urinary sodium excretion were suppressed to the same degree during renal artery constriction regardless of whether an adrenergic blocking agent was infused.

TABLE 4

Effects of Renal Artery Constriction and Adrenergic

	Number of Experiments	RVRA (ng/100ml)	Arterial PRA (ng/100ml)	Renal Blood Flow (ml/min)
Control		266.7±31.5	267.4±28.1	174.1±66.5
Constriction	7	435.0±71.7[a]	314.4±58.1	98.6±62.7
Recovery		288.1±38.3[a]	274.0±39.3	148.0±79.1
Control		274.6±40.3	258.8±29.8	178.8±46.5
Constriction + Phentolamine (8.8µg/kg/min)	8	256.8±29.2	253.2±24.9	65.6±49.6[b]
Recovery		257.4±42.6	253.8±31.2	172.0±56.2[c]
Control		285.6±45.1	281.5±47.5	253.3±157.6
Constriction + Propranolol (2µg/kg/min)	5	283.8±43.0	274.8±37.3	119.9±72.7[c]
Recovery		259.0±23.0	255.3±23.7	242.8±178.6

Values are means ± SD.
[a] p 0.001
[b] p 0.005 (constriction compared to control or recovery)
[c] p 0.05

Blockers on Renin and Renal Hemodynamics

Renin Secretion (ng/min)	Creatinine Clearance (ml/min)	Urine Flow (ml/min)	Urine Na$^+$ Excretion (µEq/min)	Heart Rate (beats/min)	Arterial B.P. (mm Hg)
17.1±13.8	22.9±10.4	0.65±0.2	112.9±49.4	136.9±12.1	108.9±11.8
138.2±128.6[c]	11.9±8.0[c]	0.32±0.2[c]	52.3±32.5[c]	146.3±16.9	111.6±14.5
22.4±11.6[c]	22.2±9.8[c]	0.58±0.2[c]	110.8±31.5[b]	144.6±20.5	107.9±18.7
26.1±12.7	20.2±11.4	0.64±0.2	92.5±44.6	140.8±17.1	115.8±15.4
4.8±2.1[b]	14.9±5.5[b]	0.30±0.1[b]	39.7±24.7[c]	139.6±9.6	110.0±18.5
18.8±13.4[c]	29.1±10.7[c]	0.63±0.2[c]	93.8±41.9[c]	138.4±16.4	113.2±14.9
28.3±33.8	29.4±12.2	0.51±0.3	79.3±50.4	142.0±15.4	112.8±22.6
15.9±16.9	11.2±5.8[c]	0.28±0.2[c]	45.6±35.7	138.0±15.9	115.0±17.3
33.9±45.0	26.9±12.8[c]	0.56±0.2[b]	70.1±41.3	141.5±13.0	112.5±17.1

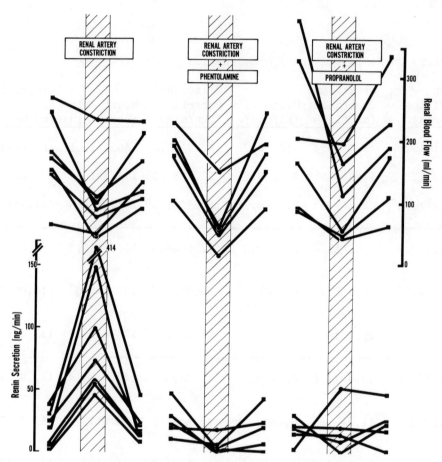

Figure 5. Effects of renal artery constriction and adrenergic
           blocking agents on renin secretion and renal blood
           flow. Squares represent control periods and circles
           represent periods of renal artery constriction.
           Enhanced renin secretion was prevented by infusion
           of either phentolamine or propranolol, while the
           reduced renal blood flow was unaffected.

significant changes in either RVRA or arterial PRA, despite the
fact that renal blood flow fell from 178.8 ± 46.5 to 65.6 ± 49.6ml
per minute during clamping (p < 0.005) and then rose during the
recovery period to 172.0 ± 56.2ml per minute (p < 0.05). Indeed,
the calculated mean renin secretion during administration of phentolamine decreased from 26.1 ± 12.7 to 4.8 ± 2.1ng per minute
(p < 0.005) and then rose to 18.8 ± 13.4ng per minute (p < 0.05).
In parallel with the fall in renal blood flow,glomerular filtration
rate, urine flow and urine sodium excretion also declined. However,
no significant differences were observed in mean heart rate or mean
arterial blood pressure during phentolamine infusion.

Similarly, the infusion of propranolol, 2μg per kg per minute,
via the femoral vein was associated with no significant change in
either RVRA or arterial PRA, despite a reduction in renal blood
flow from 253.3 ± 157.6 to 119.9 ± 72.7ml per minute (p < 0.05).
Moreover, mean renin secretion declined from 28.3 ± 33.8 to 15.9 ±
16.9ng per minute and rose during the recovery period to 33.9 ±
45.0ng per minute. These changes, however, were not significant.
The decrease in renal blood flow was accompanied by a diminution in
creatinine clearance, urine flow and urine sodium excretion during
renal artery constriction-propranolol infusion. Mean heart rate
and mean arterial blood pressure remained constant during renal
artery constriction and propranolol infusion.

DISCUSSION

It is generally considered that there are four major factors
which are capable of causing release of renin from the kidney:
1) a decrease in the pressure or tension exerted on the juxtaglomerular cells in the media of the afferent arterioles, 2) a decrease in the sodium load reaching the macula densa segment of the
distal tubule, 3) increased activity of the sympathetic nervous
system, and 4) elevated levels of circulating catecholamines. The
stimuli used in the present investigation act by one or more of the
above mechanisms to provoke an increase in renin secretion. The
data presented confirm previous observations that stimuli such as
acute hemorrhage (5,6,7), adrenalectomy (8,9), chronic salt depletion (10,11,12), and renal artery constriction (13,14) give rise to
enhanced renin secretion. The present findings indicate, in
addition, that the augmentation of renin secretion resulting from
each of these stimuli can be completely suppressed by administration
of either an α or β adrenergic blocking agent.
Acute hemorrhage has been shown to increase the release of
renin in dogs (5), rabbits (6) and rats (7). The mechanism of the
increased renin production is thought to be related to the reduction
in blood pressure following blood loss which leads to a decrease in
renal arterial perfusion pressure, a relaxation of the tension of
the afferent arteriolar walls in which the juxtaglomerular cells

are located, and consequent renin release. In addition, cardiovascular reflexes, initiated by reduced systemic blood pressure,
might also have stimulated the release of renin by enhancing
sympathetic nervous system activity and/or release of catecholamines,
since acute blood loss resulted in a significant reduction of mean
arterial blood pressure both in rats receiving phentolamine or
propranolol and untreated rats. Thus, the failure of hemorrhage to
produce the expected rise of PRA in phentolamine and propranolol-
treated rats cannot be attributed to any effect of the adrenergic
antagonists on blood pressure. Also, acute hemorrhage might have
stimulated renin secretion by decreasing renal blood flow and
delivery of sodium to the macula densa region of the distal tubule.
While sodium excretion was not measured during hemorrhage, the
possibility that the adrenergic blocking agents might somehow have
affected the sodium excretion would seem unlikely in view of their
failure to affect sodium excretion in dogs during renal artery
constriction. Finally, it is possible that the adrenergic antagonists may have affected the renin response to acute hemorrhage by
blocking the effects of catecholamines on adrenergic receptor sites
in the kidney.

As shown in the present study, chronic adrenal insufficiency in
humans (9) and in rats (8) consistently increases PRA and also renal
renin content and juxtaglomerular cell granulation (8). Most studies
indicate that increased renin secretion in adrenocortical insufficiency is due to a diminution in total body sodium concentration
rather than a deficiency in the negative feed back effect of
aldosterone on renin release, since therapy of primary aldosteronism
with spironolactone causes an increase in plasma renin concentration
(11) and administration of exogenous aldosterone in the sodium
depleted state is insufficient to reduce increased PRA (15), whereas,
the decreased juxtaglomerular cell granulation caused by desoxycorti-
costerone acetate administration is prevented by reducing the sodium
intake (16). Our data indicate that adrenalectomized rats had a
significant reduction in blood pressure compared to control rats.
With propranolol administration, the rise of PRA in adrenalectomized
rats was prevented despite the fact that blood pressure was similar
to that of untreated adrenalectomized rats. The role of the sympathetic nervous system or release of catecholamines in stimulating
renin secretion is uncertain, since there was no increase in heart
rate in adrenalectomized rats, as compared with the control group,
nor did β blockade significantly decrease the heart rate in adrenalectomized animals.

Sodium depletion resulting from deprivation of dietary sodium
has been shown to increase PRA in humans (10,11,12) and dogs (16,19)
and increase renal renin content in rats (22,23). It has also been
observed in dogs receiving a low salt diet that the increase in PRA
is not accompanied by significant changes in mean arterial blood
pressure, renal plasma flow, glomerular filtration rate, or plasma

sodium concentration (20). The present studies, in agreement with
observations made by others, showed no change in mean arterial
blood pressure in rats subjected to 7 days of a sodium deficient
diet, nor did changes in blood pressure occur with doses of phentolamine or propranolol which completely prevented the rise in PRA
induced by a low salt diet. On the other hand, salt depletion was
probably associated with increased sympathetic nervous system
activity and/or catecholamine release, since propronolol administration significantly reduced mean heart rate in rats receiving low
salt intake. Thus, our findings are consistent with the observations of Gordon et al (21) that a salt deficient diet increases
catecholamine excretion and PRA and suggest that the effect of
adrenergic blocking agents in suppressing the sodium deprivation-
induced rise in PRA may be to interfere with the action of catecholamines, although it would be unusual for <u>both</u> α and β adrenergic
antagonists to have an inhibitory effect.

    Renal artery constriction would appear to increase renin sec-
retion by a purely intrarenal mechanism, since neither systemic
blood pressure or heart rate changed during acute renal artery
constriction. It is apparent that renal blood flow, glomerular
filtration rate, and urinary sodium excretion were significantly
decreased during clamping of the renal artery. Thus, either the
renal baroreceptors or the distal tubular macula densa cells must
have been playing a role in the enhanced renin secretion. The
suppressive effect of phentolamine and propranolol administration
during the periods of renal artery constriction were apparent only
on renin secretion, whereas, the reduction of renal blood flow,
glomerular filtration rate and urinary sodium excretion was as great
or greater during administration of adrenergic antagonists. These
findings indicate that the inhibition of renin secretion during
administration of adrenergic blocking agents is independent of renal
hemodynamics. Moreover, the increase in RVRA during renal artery
constriction did not result from an increase in renin concentration
secondary to a reduction of renal blood flow. The rise observed in
arterial PRA during clamping, moreover, also favors the interpretation that renin production by the kidney was increased.

    We have previously shown that phentolamine and propranolol are
capable of suppressing the rise in plasma renin activity provoked
by upright posture and the administration of diazoxide, ethacrynic
acid, and theophylline (1), agents which have been shown to inhibit
cyclic nucleotide phosphodiesterase activity (22). In addition,
renal artery infusion of cyclic AMP also increases renin secretion,
an effect which is also inhibited by either phentolamine or propranolol infusion (2). These observations suggest that phentolamine and
propranolol may inhibit renin secretion at an intracellular site
distal to cyclic AMP production, rather than at classical adrenergic
receptor sites. The findings in the present study indicate that
both acute and chronic stimuli to renin secretion, in addition to

physiologic and pharmacologic stimuli (1), are inhibited by
adrenergic antagonists. The diverse nature of the stimuli that are
inhibited by adrenergic blockers raises the possibility that many,
if not all, stimuli of renin secretion act through a common pathway.
In view of the evidence that the inhibitory site of the adrenergic
blockers is beyond cyclic AMP production, it is likely that the
cyclic nucleotide is an intermediary along this pathway. The role
of cyclic AMP as a mediator of renin secretion is currently being
investigated.

ACKNOWLEDGEMENTS

This investigation was supported by the Kansas City Heart
Association and the Woolford Foundation of Kansas City.

REFERENCES

1.   Winer, N., Chokshi, D.S., Yoon, M.S. and Freedman, A.D.:
          Adrenergic receptor mediation of renin secretion. J. Clin.
          Endocrinol. 29:1168, 1969.
2.   Winer, N., Chokshi, D.S. and Walkenhorst, W.G.: Effects of
          cyclic AMP, sympathomimetic amines and adrenergic antag-
          onists on renin secretion. Circulation Res. 29:239,1971.
3.   Hartroft, P.M. and Eisenstein, A.B.: Alterations in the
          adrenal cortex of the rat induced by sodium deficiency:
          correlation of histologic changes with steroid hormone
          secretion. Endocrinol. 60:641, 1957.
4.   Gunnels, J.C., Grim, C.E., Robinson, R.R. and Wilderman, N.M.:
          Plasma renin activity in healthy subjects and patients with
          hypertension. Arch. Int. Med. 119:232, 1967.
5.   Huidobro, F. and Braun-Menendez, E.: The secretion of renin by
          the intact kidney. Am. J. Physiolog. 137:47, 1942.
6.   McKenzie, J.K., Cook, W.F. and Lee, M.R.: Effect of haemorrhage
          on arterial plasma renin activity in the rabbit. Circula-
          tion Res. 19:269, 1966.
7.   Ziegler, M. and Gross, F.: Effect of blood volume changes on
          renin-like activity in blood. Proc. Soc. Exper. Biol. &
          Med. 116:774, 1964.
8.   Sokabe, H., Mikasa, A., Yasuda, H. and Masson, G.M.C.:
          Adrenal cortex and renal pressor function. Circulation
          Res. 12:94, 1963.
9.   Brown, J.J., Davies, D.L., Lever, A.F. and Robertson, J.I.S.:
          Variations in plasma renin concentration in several
          physiological and pathological states. Canad. M.A.J. 90:
          201, 1964.
10.   Fasciolo, J.C., DeVito, E., Romero, J.C. and Cucchi, J.N.:
          The renin content of the blood of humans and dogs under
          several conditions. Canad. M.A.J. 90:206, 1964.

11. Brown, J.J., Davies, D.L., Lever, A.F. and Robertson, J.I.S.:
        Influence of sodium deprivation and loading on plasma renin
        in man. J.Physiol. 173:408, 1964.
12. Ajzen, H., Simmons, J.L. and Woods, J.W.: Renal vein renin and
        juxtaglomerular activity in sodium-depleted subjects.
        Circulation Res. 17:130, 1965.
13. Skinner, S.L., McCubbin, J.W. and Page, I.H.: Renal baro-
        receptor control of acute renin release in normotensive,
        nephrogenic and neurogenic hypertensive dogs. Circulation
        Res. 15:522, 1964.
14. Lever, A.F., Robertson, J.I.S. and Tree, M.: The assay of renin
        in rabbit plasma. In Hormones and the Kidney, p. 285.
        Ed. Williams, P., Academic Press, New York, 1963.
15. Genest, J., de Champlain, J., Veyrat, R., Boucher, R.,
        Tremblay, G.Y., Strong, C.G., Koiw, E. and Marc-Aurele, J.:
        Role of the renin-angiotensin system in various physiologi-
        cal and pathological states. Hypertension 13:97, 1965.
16. Hartroft, P.M.: Histological and functional aspects of juxta-
        glomerular cells, in Angiotensin Systems and Experimental
        Renal Diseases. Ed. Metcoff, Little, Brown & Co., Boston,
        1963.
17. Scornik, O.A. and Paladini, A.C.: Significance of blood
        angiotensin levels in different experimental conditions.
        Canad. M.A.J. 90:269, 1964.
18. Binnion, P.F., Davis, J.O., Brown, T.C., Olichney, M.J.:
        Mechanisms regulating aldosterone secretion during sodium
        depletion. Am. J. Physiol. 208:655, 1965.
19. Gross, F., Brunner, H. and Ziegler, M.: Renin-angiotensin
        system, aldosterone and sodium balance. Recent Prog.
        Hormone Res. 21:119, 1965.
20. Brubacher, E.S. and Vander, A.J.: Sodium deprivation and renin
        secretion in unanesthetized dogs. Fed. Proc. 25:432, 1966.
21. Gordon, R.D., Kuchel, O., Liddle G.W. and Island, D.P.: Role
        of the sympathetic nervous system in regulating renin and
        aldosterone production in man. J.Clin. Invest. 46:599, 1967
22. Winer, N. and Chaudhuri, T.K.: Effect of renin-stimulating
        agents on renal cortical phosphodiesterase activity.
        Clin. Res. 18:601, 1970.

RENIN SECRETION, ADRENERGIC BLOCKADE AND HYPERTENSION

A.M. Michelakis and R.G. McAllister, Jr.

Departments of Medicine and Pharmacology, Vanderbilt

University School of Medicine, Nashville, Tennessee

In the last few years, considerable effort has been made by several investigators to elucidate the mechanism that regulates renin secretion. Initially, attention was directed at testing either the macula densa theory or the baroreceptor hypothesis. There is evidence, however, that the sympathetic nervous system is also involved. Both in vitro (1) and organ perfusion (2) studies have demonstrated that catecholamines will increase renin secretion from the kidney. In addition, intravenous infusion of catecholamines to normal man markedly increased plasma renin activity (PRA) (3), and recent work in dogs has shown that intravenous infusion of isoproterenol increased PRA (4).

Recent studies have shown that infusion of either alpha (phentolamine) or beta (propranolol) adrenergic blockers to normal subjects, acutely blocked the renin rise after standing (5). These agents also blocked the PRA rise after diazoxide, ethacrynic acid, or theophylline administration (5). In other studies (6) performed in dogs, it was found that the rise of renin secretion with epinephrine was abolished with propranolol, while it was potentiated with phenoxybenzamine.

In the present study we investigated the effect of chronic oral administration of phenoxybenzamine and propranolol on supine and upright PRA in hypertensive patients under well controlled conditions of posture and sodium intake and the results are reported here.

83

METHODS

Three normal volunteers and ten hypertensive patients were studied. Five patients had essential hypertension, three had significant unilateral renal artery stenosis, and two had bilateral renal artery stenosis. All medications were discontinued for at least two weeks prior to their hospitalization in the Clinical Research Center. The subjects were given 100 or 10 mEq sodium diets and the study begun when they were in sodium balance. Blood pressure was measured in the supine and standing position every six hours.

After the subjects had been in sodium balance on 100 mEq sodium diet for at least three days, supine and upright PRA was measured. Subjects were supine for the entire eight-hour period preceding the supine (8AM) determination, subsequently they assumed the upright position for the next three hours and PRA was measured at 9,10, and 11 AM. They were begun the following day on oral propranolol 20 mg every six hours and PRA measurements were repeated after 72 hours of drug administration. Subjects were then brought into sodium balance on a 10 mEq sodium diet and the same protocol repeated. Response of PRA to increasing doses of propranolol was also studied in four patients.

The effect of phenoxybenzamine on PRA was studied in four of the hypertensive patients (two with essential hypertension, one with bilateral renal artery stenosis, and one with unilateral significant renal artery stenosis) while they were in balance on the 10 mEq sodium diet. Supine and upright control blood samples for PRA determination were obtained from each patient. Subsequently, they were given phenoxybenzamine 10 mg every twelve hours for four days and then PRA was determined as before.

In a patient with renovascular hypertension, recumbent and upright PRA was measured while he was in sodium balance on 10 mEq sodium diet. He was studied while on placebo for six days and again after six days of oral propranolol 30 mg every six hours.

PRA was measured by known procedures (7,8). The possibility that either propranolol or phenoxybenzamine might interfere with the assay of renin was excluded by showing that addition of excess of these substances to plasma samples did not affect renin levels.

RESULTS

Pooled data on the effect of chronic propranolol administration 20 mg every six hours are shown in Figure 1. In all subjects beta-adrenergic blockade produced a fall in PRA, both in the supine and the standing positions. Total suppression of renin with

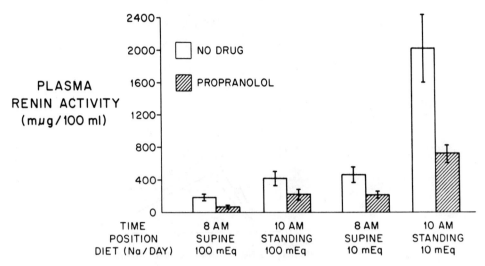

Figure 1.   The effect of oral propranolol, 80 mg per day for 3
            days, upon plasma renin activity (mean $\pm$ SE) in the
            supine and standing positions and on 100 and 10 mEq
            sodium diets.   Data are from both normotensive and
            hypertensive subjects.   Propranolol significantly
            suppressed PRA in each category ($p < 0.05$).

propranolol was not seen in any subject.   It is of interest that
the expected rise in PRA after standing and sodium deprivation
was not eliminated but it was only blunted.   The effects of varying oral doses of propranolol on PRA in the supine position and
after standing for one, two, and three hours in a patient with
essential hypertension and in a patient with renovascular hypertension while on 10 mEq sodium daily are shown in Figures 2 and
3, respectively.   As the dose of propranolol increased, PRA levels
fell at each point in time.

Significant supine or upright blood pressure fall was not seen
in any subject while they were on low doses of propranolol. A
significant reduction of blood pressure, however, was noted in a
patient who received 160 and 320 mg propranolol per day.   Resting
pulse fell significantly in all normal subjects and in four hypertensive patients.

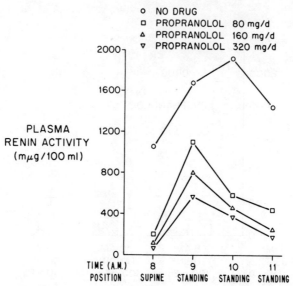

Figure 2.   The effect of varying doses of propranolol on plasma
            renin activity in the supine position and after one,
            two, and three hours standing in a patient with
            essential hypertension while in balance on 10 mEq
            sodium daily.

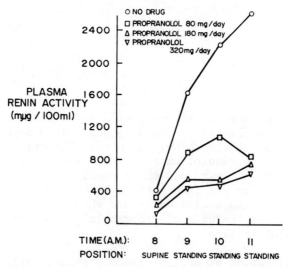

Figure 3.   The effect of varying oral doses of propranolol on
            plasma renin activity in the supine position and after
            one, two, and three hours standing in a patient with
            renovascular hypertension while in balance on a diet
            containing 10 mEq sodium daily.

The changes in blood pressure, pulse rate, and plasma renin activity in a patient with renovascular hypertension who received 30 mg propranolol every six hours for six days while he was in balance on 10 mEq sodium diet are shown in Figure 4. Although the changes in mean daily supine and upright blood pressure between the placebo and propranolol periods were not statistically significant, there was a marked fall in PRA.

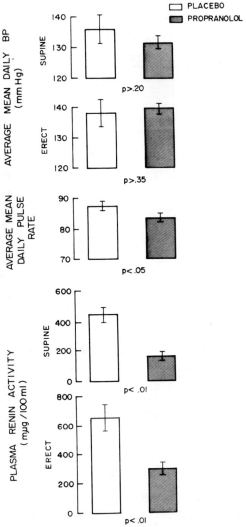

Figure 4. The effect of oral propranolol 30 mg every six hours for six days, upon blood pressure, pulse rate, and plasma renin activity (mean + SE) in a patient with renovascular hypertension while in balance on 10 mEq sodium daily.

The combined data on the effect of phenoxybenzamine, 10 mg
every twelve hours for four days, on supine and standing PRA are
shown in Figure 5. In all subjects studied there was little or
no change in PRA with phenoxybenzamine. A postural drop in blood
pressure with phenoxybenzamine was seen in all subjects. There
was no substantial effect on supine blood pressure or resting
pulse rate.

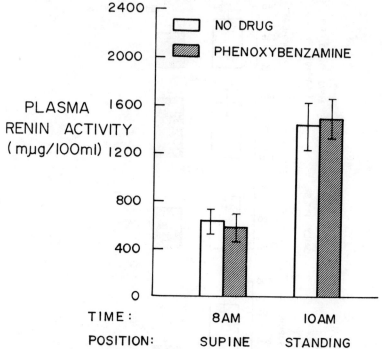

Figure 5.   Response of supine and standing plasma renin activity
            (mean + SE) to alpha-adrenergic blockade with phenoxy-
            benzamine in hypertensive patients. All studies were
            carried out on a diet containing 10 mEq sodium per
            day.

DISCUSSION

Previous studies with normal individuals (5) have shown that
alpha or beta receptor blockade would acutely suppress the PRA
rise caused by various stimuli. Other investigators (9) found that
stimulation of renin secretion could be prevented with propranolol
but not with phentolamine. Similarly, other investigators (6)
found that, in dogs, beta-blockade with propranolol prevented the
rise of renin during hypoglycemia, whereas alpha-blockade with
phenoxybenzamine did not inhibit the renin rise. We performed

our studies with normal subjects and patients with essential and
renovascular hypertension. Our results along with those of others
(5,9,6) provide evidence that beta-adrenergic receptors predominate
in regulating renin secretion. Relying on endogenous stimuli,
we have shown that chronic beta-adrenergic blockade caused significant renin suppression in both sodium excess and sodium depletion
as well as in both the supine and standing positions. Alpha-
adrenergic blockade with phenoxybenzamine was not similarly effective. Although beta-adrenergic receptors may play an important
role in renin secretion, the rise in PRA with upright posture and
sodium depletion was not totally inhibited by beta-blockade.
This supports the view that other factors independent of adrenergic
mechanisms may also be involved in the control of renin secretion.

Since Goldblatt's classic experiments in which he showed that
renal artery constriction caused hypertension (10), many investigators believe that an increase of renin release from the ischemic
kidney is the cause of renovascular hypertension. Some patients,
however, with renovascular hypertension do not always have elevated
plasma renin levels (11,12). Further, experimental renovascular
hypertension could be developed in rabbits which were pre-immunized
with angiotensin II (13). Similarly, immunization of hypertensive
rabbits against angiotensin (14) did not lower blood pressure.
It is possible, therefore, that the renin-angiotensin system may
not be the primary factor in the pathogenesis of renovascular
hypertension. In the present study this possibility was also
investigated. With low doses of propranolol, there was little or
no change in blood pressure although there was a significant drop
in PRA. A representative study in a patient with renovascular
hypertension is shown in Figure 4. There was little or no change
in blood pressure with chronic propranolol administration in spite
of a marked drop in supine and standing PRA. These findings support the view that renin may not be the sole factor in the etiology of renovascular hypertension and that some other factors may
be involved.

SUMMARY

Plasma renin activity was measured in human subjects before
and after chronic alpha-adrenergic blockade with phenoxybenzamine
and beta blockade with propranolol under well controlled conditions
of posture and diet. The rise of PRA with upright posture and sodium deprivation was partially but significantly suppressed in all
subjects with propranolol but not with phenoxybenzamine. The
findings suggest that, under these experimental conditions, the
beta and not the alpha receptors play an important role on renin
release and that other factors should also be considered in its
secretion. The suppression of supine and upright PRA with beta-
adrenergic blockade was not accompanied by decrease in blood

pressure suggesting that, in addition to renin, other factors are involved in the pathogenesis of renovascular hypertension.

ACKNOWLEDGEMENTS

The research described was supported by U.S. Public Health Service grants HE12683, GM 15431, and HE05545.

REFERENCES

1. Michelakis, A.M., Caudle, J., and Liddle, G.W.: In vitro stimulation of renin production by epinephrine, norepinephrine and cyclic AMP. Proc Soc Exp Biol Med 130:748, 1969.
2. Vander, A.J.: Effect of catecholamines and the renal nerves on renin secretion in anesthetized dogs. Am J Physiol 209:659, 1965.
3. Michelakis, A.M. and Horton, R.: The relationship between plasma renin and aldosterone in normal man. Circulation Res (suppl) 27:I-185, 1970.
4. Wallace, J.M., Andersen, F.G., and Sheppard, H.A., Jr.: Beta-adrenergic stimulation of renin secretion. Clin Res 28:28, 1970.
5. Winer, N., Chokshi, D.S., Yoon, M.S., and Freedman, A.D.: Adrenergic receptor mediation of renin secretion. J Clin Endocr 29:1168, 1969.
6. Assaykeen, T.A., Clayton, P.L., Goldfien, A., and Ganong, W.F.: Effect of alpha and beta-adrenergic blocking agents on the renin response to hypoglycemia and epinephrine in dogs. Endocrinology 87:1318, 1970.
7. Boucher, R., Veyrat, R., DeChamplain, J., and Genest, J.: New procedures for measurement of human plasma angiotensin and renin levels. Canad Med Assoc J 90:194, 1964.
8. Haber, E., Koerner, T., Page, L.B., Kliman, B., and Purnode,A.: Application of a radioimmunoassay for angiotensin I to the physiologic measurements of plasma renin activity in normal human subjects. J Clin Endocr 29:1349, 1969.
9. Meurer, K.A., Dieter, H.M., Schmid, D., Schmidt, H.J., and Kaufman, W.: Role of beta-adrenergic receptors in renin libera-tion. Deutsch Med Wschr 99:749, 1971.
10. Goldblatt, H., Lynch, J., Hanzal, R.F., and Summerville, W.W.: Studies on experimental hypertension. I. The production of per-sistent elevation of systolic blood pressure by means of renal ischemia. J Exper Med 59:347, 1934.
11. Laragh, J.H., Sealey, J.E., and Sommers, S.C.: Patterns of adrenal secretion and urinary excretion of aldosterone and plasma renin activity in normal and hypertensive subjects. Circulation Res 18: Suppl. I, 158, 1966.

12. Mulrow, P.J., Lytton, B., and Stansel, H.C.: The role of the
     renin angiotensin system in the hypertension associated with
     renal vascular disease. In L'Hypertension Arterielle, ed.
     by Milliez and P. Tcherdakoff, L'Expansion Scientifique
     Francaise, Paris, 1966.
13. Mcdonald, G.J., Louis, W.J., Renzini, V., Boyd, G.W., and
     Peart, W.S.: Renal clip hypertension in rabbits immunized
     against angiotensin II. Circulation Res 27:197, 1970.
14. Johnston, C.I., Hutchinson, J.S. and Mendelsohn, F.A.:
     Biological significance of renin angiotensin immunization.
     Circulation Res 26&27: Suppl II, 215, 1970.

STUDIES ON THE MECHANISM OF RENIN SUPPRESSION BY ALPHA-METHYLDOPA

P.J. Privitera and S. Mohammed

Division of Clinical Pharmacology, Departments of

Medicine and Pharmacology, University of Cincinnati

College of Medicine, Cincinnati, Ohio

Recent observations from this laboratory made in human subjects on chronic methyldopa treatment indicate that this antihypertensive drug produces a decrease in plasma renin activity simultaneously with a reduction in mean arterial pressure (Mohammed et al., 1969). Methyldopa reduced plasma renin activity in both the supine and tilted positions in these subjects (Figure 1). This suppressive effect of methyldopa treatment on the renin-angiotensin system has subsequently been confirmed in a child with Bartter's syndrome who had markedly elevated plasma renin activity (Strauss et al., 1970). This effect of methyldopa is contrary to that observed with other antihypertensive agents. For example, hydralazine (Ueda et al., 1968) diazoxide (Kuchel et al., 1967) and reserpine (Ayers et al., 1968) are all reported to increase plasma renin activity in normotensive or hypertensive subjects or dogs.

The present studies performed in adult dogs were undertaken to clarify the possible mechanisms responsible for the suppression of renin release produced by chronic treatment with methyldopa.

Effect of Methyldopa on Plasma Renin Activity in Dogs

Our initial studies established that chronic treatment with methyldopa was associated with a reduction in plasma renin activity in dogs (Mohammed and Privitera, 1971). Blood samples for plasma renin activity determinations were analyzed by a modified method (Brubacher and Vander, 1968) of Boucher and associates (1964). Sodium content of the diet was not controlled. Plasma renin activity in eleven control dogs was 13.09 ± 2.02 ng/ml of formed angiotensin per 3 hr incubation. In eight dogs pretreated with oral methyldopa, 200 mg/kg/day for 7 to 10 days, plasma renin

93

activity was 7.31 ± 1.12; this value was significantly less
(p < 0.05) than that observed for the control group (Figure 2).
The foregoing results indicate that the dog is a suitable animal
in which to study the suppressive effect of methyldopa on the
renin-angiotensin system.

Effect of Methyldopa on Renin Release produced by Renal Nerve Stimulation

The sympathetic nervous system exerts an important influence
over the control of renin secretion by the kidney. Direct electrical
stimulation of the renal nerves produces marked increases in plasma
renin activity (Vander, 1965). In addition, the administration of
catecholamines has also been observed to increase renin release from
the kidney (Vander, 1965; Bunag et al., 1966).

A logical approach to the definition of the factors involved in
the suppression of renin by methyldopa was to examine the influence
of methyldopa on the release of renin produced by sympathetic nerve
stimulation. In this series of experiments in pentobarbital-
anesthetized dogs, the left renal artery was cannulated and perfused
with blood from the femoral artery. Blood flow to the kidney was
measured with an electromagnetic flowmeter using a cannulating flow
probe. Electrodes were placed on the renal nerves to the left
kidney. The kidney was denervated by cutting all visible renal nerve
fibers central to the electrode and by applying 95% phenol solution
on the nerves and surrounding tissue. This was done to eliminate
changes in plasma renin activity that might occur due to changes in
sympathetic tone to the kidney. A diagram of the renal perfusion
technique is presented in Figure 3. The left renal nerve was stimulated at a frequency of 10 cps with the stimulation voltage adjusted
to produce a 50% reduction in renal blood flow.

Plasma renin activity was significantly increased (p < 0.001)
after 20 minutes of renal nerve stimulation in the control group of
animals. In dogs chronically treated with methyldopa, however,
renal nerve stimulation produced no significant increase in plasma
renin activity (p < 0.1; Figure 4). These results indicate that
chronic treatment with methyldopa can impair the release of renin
produced by renal sympathetic nerve stimulation. This impairment
was not produced by adrenergic neuronal blockade of the renal
sympathetic nerves by methyldopa since renal nerve stimulation
produced the same magnitude of renal vasoconstriction in the control
and methyldopa-treated animals. The absence of an increase in
plasma renin levels despite an increase in renal vascular resistance
in methyldopa-treated dogs, is consistent with the hypothesis that
renin secretion induced by nerve stimulation is not secondary to
renal afferent arteriolar constriction but is related to a direct
action of the catecholamines on the renin-producing cells (Michelakis
et al., 1969), presumably through a beta-receptor mechanism (Passo

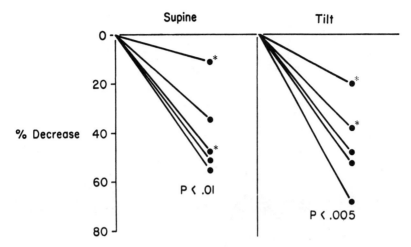

Figure 1. The effect of oral methyldopa on plasma renin activity
in one hypertensive and four normotensive subjects in
supine and tilted positions.

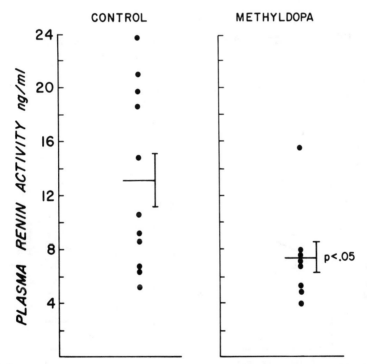

Figure 2. The effect of pretreatment with oral methyldopa on
plasma renin activity in anesthetized dogs. Vertical
bars indicate 1 S.E.M.

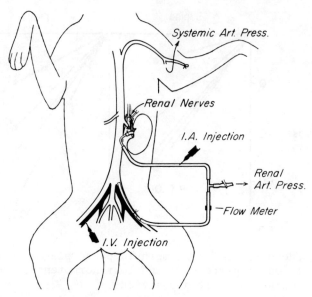

Figure 3.   Renal perfusion scheme.

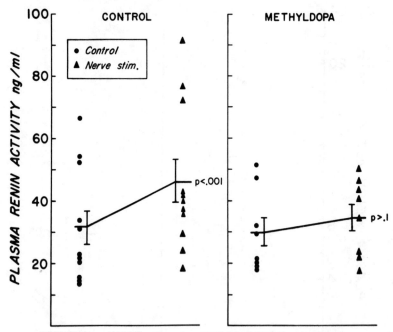

Figure 4.   Effect of renal nerve stimulation on plasma renin
            activity in 11 control dogs and 8 dogs pretreated
            with oral methyldopa, 200 mg/kg/day for 7 to 10 days.

et al., 1971).

It is well known that treatment with methyldopa leads to displacement in nerve endings of the natural transmitter, norepinephrine
with "false" transmitter alpha-methylnorepinephrine. This amine
metabolite of methyldopa replaces norepinephrine in the nerve endings
on an equimolar basis and can be released by adrenergic nerve stimulation (Carlsson and Lindqvist, 1962; Maitre and Staehelin, 1963).
The possibility was considered that in animals treated with methyldopa, the methylnorepinephrine stored in the renal sympathetic
nerves and released with nerve stimulation is less potent than
norepinephrine on the adrenergic receptor mediating renin release.
A decreased potency for methylnorepinephrine could account for the
insignificant rise in plasma renin activity seen with nerve stimulation in methyldopa-treated dogs.

Effect of Norepinephrine and Methylnorepinephrine on Plasma Renin Activity

In another series of animals, the effects of intravenous
infusions of norepinephrine and methylnorepinephrine on plasma renin
activity were compared in anesthetized dogs. During a 20-minute
infusion of each drug, the renal arterial pressure was held at
control level by means of an inflated balloon catheter positioned
in the aorta above both renal arteries. The order of drug infusion
was randomized. Both catecholamines infused at a rate of 11.8×10^{-3}
μM/kg/min (approximately 2 μg/kg/min), produced significant increases
in plasma renin activity during infusion (Figure 5). However, the
increase in plasma renin activity observed during norepinephrine
infusion was significantly greater ($p < 0.02$) than that observed with
methylnorepinephrine. These data support the concept that methyldopa's suppressive effect on plasma renin activity may be related to
the release of the less potent "false" transmitter, methylnorepinephrine from the renal sympathetic nerve endings.

The preceding experiments indicate that methyldopa suppresses
plasma renin activity via its effect on the sympathetic nervous
system. However, it was also necessary to consider the possibility
that methyldopa might affect plasma renin levels through a direct
action on the kidney.

Effect of Methyldopa on Renin Release in Response to Reduction in Renal Arterial Pressure in the Acutely Denervated Kidney.

In this series of experiments, perfusion pressure to the
denervated left kidneys of four control and four methyldopa-treated
dogs was reduced 50 mm Hg by occluding the renal perfusion tubing
with an adjustable clamp (Figure 3). During occlusion, plasma

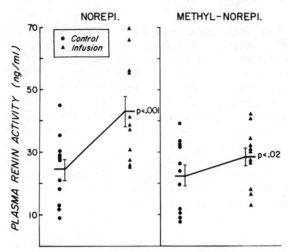

Figure 5.   Effects of systemic intravenous infusions of
            norepinephrine and methylnorepinephrine on plasma
            renin activity in 11 control dogs. Both drugs were
            infused at a rate of 11.8 x 10^{-3} µM/kg/min in
            each dog.

renin activity increased equally in both groups as illustrated in
Figure 6. These results demonstrate that chronic methyldopa treatment does not impair the kidney's ability to release renin in
response to decreased perfusion pressure.

Effect of Methyldopa on Renal Vascular Resistance in the Dog

During the course of our studies it was observed that renal
vascular resistance in the denervated kidney was significantly less
(p < 0.05) in dogs pretreated with methyldopa as compared to control
dogs (Figure 7). Methyldopa has previously been reported to significantly reduce renal vascular resistance in patients with essential
hypertension in both the supine and tilted positions (Mohammed et
al., 1968). The decreased renal vascular resistance produced by
methyldopa may occur as a result of impaired renin release since it
is seen in the denervated as well as the innervated kidney.

Effect of Norepinephrine and Methylnorepinephrine on
Renal Vascular Resistance in Dogs

Methylnorepinephrine was also found to be a less potent vasoconstrictor than norepinephrine in the renal vasculature. Comparison
of responses to injections of these two agents into the renal artery

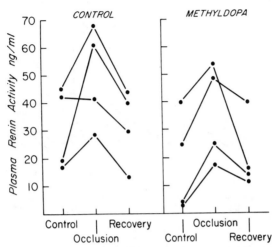

Figure 6.   The effect of reduction in renal arterial pressure on
plasma renin activity in 4 control and 4 methyldopa-
treated dogs (200 mg/kg/day for 7 to 10 days).

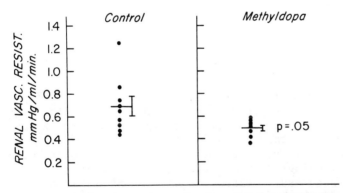

Figure 7.   The effect of pretreatment with methyldopa on renal
vascular resistance in dogs. Methyldopa-treated dogs
received 200 mg/kg/day of drug for 7 to 10 days.

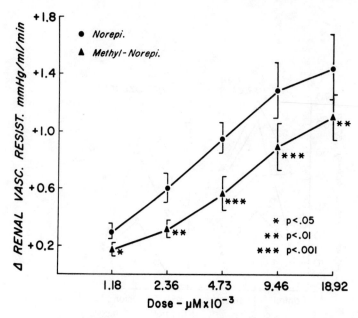

Figure 8.   The effects of intra-arterial norepinephrine and
            methylnorepinephrine on renal vascular resistance
            in 7 control dogs.

indicates that methylnorepinephrine has about one-third to one-half
the activity of norepinephrine with respect to renal pressor effects
in the dog (Figure 8).

SUMMARY

    These data indicate that chronic treatment with methyldopa
suppresses the increase in plasma renin activity associated with
renal nerve stimulation. In addition, methylnorepinephrine was
found to be less active than norepinephrine on the adrenergic
receptor mediating renin release and on the renal vascular adrenergic
receptor. These findings viewed collectively strongly support the
concept that the suppressive effect of methyldopa on plasma renin
activity is related to the displacement of norepinephrine in the
renal sympathetic nerves by a less potent "false" transmitter, alpha-
methylnorepinephrine which is formed from methyldopa.

    The increased renin release produced by local reduction in renal
arterial pressure is mediated via an intrarenal mechanism (Vander,
1967). The inability of methyldopa treatment to suppress this
response argues against a direct intrarenal action for methyldopa,
at least with respect to its effect on plasma renin activity.

ACKNOWLEDGEMENTS

This work was supported in part by U.S.P.H.S. Grants HE-12861 and HE-07392.

REFERENCES

Ayers, C.R., Harris, R.H. and Lefer, L.G.: Control of renin release in experimental hypertension. Circulation Res. 24: Suppl. I, I-103, 1969.

Boucher, R., Veyrat, R., De Champlain, J. and Genest, J.: New procedure for measurement of human plasma angiotensin and renin activity levels. Canad. Med. Assoc. J. 90:194, 1964.

Brubacher, E.S. and Vander, A.J.: Sodium deprivation and renin secretion in unanesthetized dogs. Am. J. Physiol. 214:15, 1968.

Bunag, R., Rage, I.H. and McCubbin, J.W.: Neural stimulation of release of renin. Circulation Res. 19:851, 1966.

Carlsson, A. and Lindqvist, M.: In vivo decarboxylation of α-methyl DOPA and α-methyl metatyrosine. Acta Physiol. Scand. 54:87, 1962.

Kuchel, O., Fishman, L.M., Liddle, G.W. and Michelakis, A.: Effect of diazoxide on plasma renin activity in hypertensive patients. Ann. Internal Med. 67:791, 1967.

Maitre, L. and Staehelin, M.: Effect of α-methyl-DOPA on myocardial catecholamines. Experientia 19:573, 1963.

Michelakis, A.M., Caudle, J. and Liddle, G.W.: In vitro stimulation of renin production by epinephrine, norepinephrine and cyclic AMP. Proc. Soc. Exper. Biol. Med. 130:748, 1969.

Mohammed, S., Fasola, A.F., Privitera, P.J., Lipicky, R.J., Martz, B.L. and Gaffney, T.E.: Effect of methyldopa on plasma renin activity in man. Circulation Res. 25:543, 1969.

Mohammed, S., Hanenson, I.B., Magenheim, H.G. and Gaffney, T.E.: The effects of alpha-methyldopa on renal function in hypertensive patients. Am. Heart J. 76:21, 1968.

Mohammed, S. and Privitera, P.J.: Effect of methyldopa on plasma renin activity in dogs. Clin. Res. 19:329, 1971.

Passo, S.S., Assaykeen, T.A., Goldfien, A. and Ganong, W.F.: Effect of α and β-adrenergic blocking agents on the increase in renin secretion produced by stimulation of the medulla oblongata in dog. Neuroendocrinology 7:97, 1971.

Strauss, R.G. Mohammed, S., Loggie, J.M.H., Schubert, W.K., Fasola, A.F. and Gaffney, T.E.: The effect of methyldopa on plasma renin activity in a child with Bartter's syndrome. J. Pediat. 77:1071, 1970.

Ueda, H., Yagi, S. and Kaneko, Y.: Hydralazine and plasma renin activity. Arch. Intern. Med. 122:387, 1968.

Vander, A.J.: Effect of catecholamines and the renal nerves on renin secretion in anesthetized dogs. Am. J. Physiol. 209:659, 1965.

Vander, A.J.: Control of renin release. Physiol. Rev. 47:359, 1967.

RENIN RELEASE BY VERTEBRAL ARTERY EMBOLISM

H. Ueda, Y. Uchida, A. Sakamoto and A. Ebihara

Heart Institute of Japan, Tokyo, Japan and the Second

Department of Internal Medicine, University of Tokyo,

Tokyo, Japan

It had been recently elucidated that brain stem stimulation increases renin secretion. H. Ueda and his co-workers (1) have shown that electrical stimulation of the mesencephalic pressor area (central gray stratum) in dogs increased renin release markedly and the increase was abolished by renal denervation. Passo et al (2) have found that stimulation of the medulla oblongata increased renin secretion in dogs. Blair and Feigl (3) have noticed that hypothalamic stimulation induced the increase of renin release.

On the other side, Dickinson and Yu have shown that angiotensin produces a clear pressor response by vertebral artery infusion even in low concentrations (4). In addition, we have shown that vertebral embolism enhances the blood pressure and the sympathetic nerve activity in rabbits (5,6).

The purpose of this study is to clarify the relationship between the changes of blood pressure and renin release by brain stem stimulation with vertebral artery embolism in dogs.

METHODS

Mongrel dogs anesthetized with pentobarbital sodium were used for the studies. A catheter was introduced into the left renal vein through the right femoral vein to collect the blood sample. The spermatic vein was ligated to avoid the mixing of its blood with the renal blood. One of the renal nerve bundles was transsected at the hilus and was put across the bipolar electrodes to lead off the action potentials. The efferent impulses were converted into square waves by a pulse generator and were integrated. The

103

integrated units were recorded simultaneously with the arterial
pressure. The renal blood flow was recorded by the probe of an
electromagnetic flowmeter attached on the left renal artery. Vertebral embolism was produced by slow injection over 15 seconds of
5 ml of air into a catheter inserted into the right vertebral artery.
The renal venous blood was collected 1, 6, 10, 20, 30, 45 and 60
minutes after embolism. Plasma renin activity was measured by the
method of Helmer and Judsen (7). Renin activity was expressed as
ng AT/ml, as renin release from the left kidney per minute (renal
plasma flow times ng AT/ml) and as percent change.

RESULTS

After vertebral embolism started, the blood pressure rose up
slightly and then rose up again markedly. Thereafter, it fell down
gradually to lower levels than the control in most experiments. In
the next stage, the blood pressure rose up slightly and then returned to control levels (Figure 1). On injecting the air into the
vertebral artery, a transient increase in renal sympathetic nerve
activity occurred, accompanied by the first rise in blood pressure.
Thereafter, a marked decrease in the activity was observed at the
stage of the second rise in pressure. Then, after the second steep
rise of blood pressure, marked increase of sympathetic nerve activity
occurred again. This increased sympathetic nerve activity persisted
on several occasions for as long as 20 minutes.

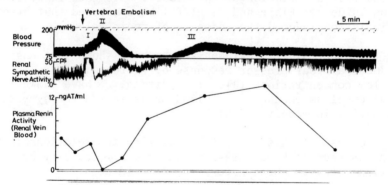

Figure 1.   The effect of vertebral embolism on blood pressure,
            renal sympathetic nerve activity and renal vein renin
            activity in a typical dog. I, II and III show the
            stages of rise in blood pressure.

The renal blood flow was reduced abruptly by air embolism and
then returned gradually to its former level. This reduction occurred concomitantly with the first rise in blood pressure. In
several experiments, a second slight reduction in renal blood flow
occurred simultaneously with the third peak in pressure (Figure 2).

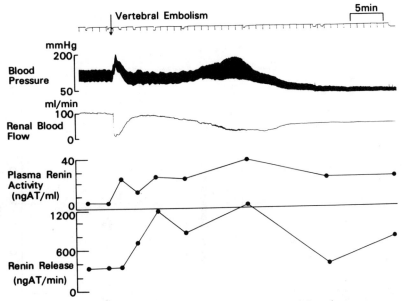

Figure 2. The effect of vertebral embolism on blood pressure,
          renal blood flow, plasma renin activity and renin
          release in a typical dog.

The plasma renin activity in control samples was 9.2 ± 4.2(mean
value ± standard deviation). One minute after the production of
embolism, plasma renin activity began to increase significantly
(p < 0.05) as shown in Figure 3. However, even when an increase in
plasma renin activity was observed following embolism, it does not
necessarily indicate an increase in renin release from the kidney.
The clear reduction in renal blood flow may have caused an apparent
increase by concentration. To clarify whether renin release from
the kidney increased, renal plasma flow (RPF) multiplied by plasma
renin activity before and after embolism was compared. Renin release from the kidney per minute thus obtained in the control phase
was 385±120 ngAT/min. It began to increase significantly ten minutes later, as shown in Figure 4.

DISCUSSION

Previously, we have observed a biphasic increase in sympathetic
discharge following vertebral embolism in rabbits. The first slight
increase in discharge accompanied the first rise in blood pressure.
Marked decrease of discharge was observed at the stage of the second
peak of pressure. Then, the second marked increase of discharge occurred after the second blood pressure peak or occasionally it coin-
cided with the third rise in blood pressure.

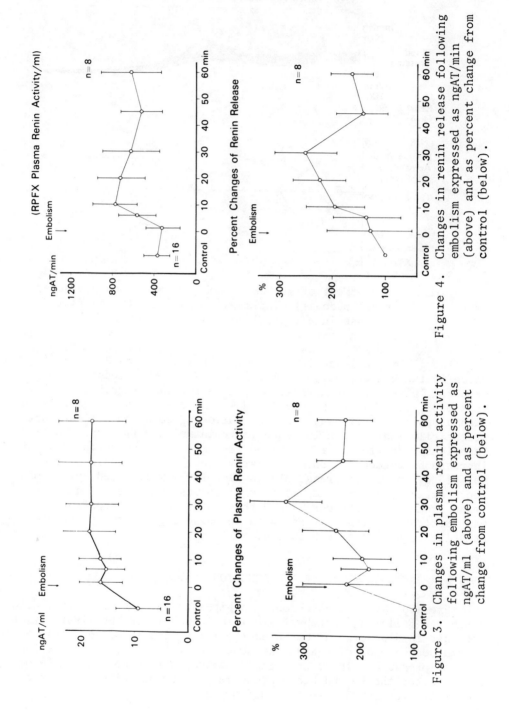

Figure 3. Changes in plasma renin activity following embolism expressed as ngAT/ml (above) and as percent change from control (below).

Figure 4. Changes in renin release following embolism expressed as ngAT/min (above) and as percent change from control (below).

After transection of the cervical vagi, aortic nerves and the carotid sinus nerves, the phase of decreased sympathetic activity became minimal or disappeared. It was considered, therefore, that the phase of reduced sympathetic activity was produced by excitation of the buffer nerves caused by the second rise in pressure. The second rise in blood pressure was not produced after administration of phenoxybenzamine and all three peaks were blocked after treatment with tetraethylammonium chloride (5,6).

The electrical stimulation of the central gray stratum of the mesencephalon in dogs caused nearly the same changes in the blood pressure, a marked increase in catecholamine release which occurred with the second rise of pressure and increased renin release which occurred about 15 minutes after the stimulation (1).

In the present experiment in dogs, vertebral embolism produced nearly the same changes in blood pressure and in sympathetic nerve activity as observed in rabbits. Renin release from the kidney began to increase after the peak of the second rise in blood pressure or just prior to the third rise in the pressure. Consequently, it is considered that the first slight rise in blood pressure caused by vertebral embolism in the present investigations was produced by the direct effect of the first sympathetic excitation on the cardiovascular system. The second rise in pressure was probably caused by the increased catecholamines which were released from the adrenal medulla. It is not likely that renin participated in these two rises in the pressure.

Three factors can be pointed out as possible mechanisms for the third rise in blood pressure: 1) increased renin, 2) increased sympathetic activity and its direct effect on the vascular system, and 3) possible increases in circulating catecholamines caused by the increased sympathetic activity. Probably all three factors are involved in the third peak in blood pressure. The fact that a marked increase in blood pressure did not accompany the marked second increase in sympathetic discharge may be attributable to decreased reactivity of the target organs.

In previous experiments involving stimulation of the central gray stratum (1), it required about 15 minutes to cause an increase in renin release. Therefore, it is more reasonable to consider that the first and not the second increase in renal nerve activity caused the increase in renin activity.

SUMMARY

The relations of renin release from the kidney to the changes in the renal sympathetic nerve activity, blood pressure and renal blood flow caused by vertebral artery embolism, were studied in anesthetized dogs. The blood pressure rose up in three stages, the sympathetic nerve activity increased in two stages and the renal blood flow fell abruptly by vertebral embolism. The first increase in the sympathetic activity was accompanied by the first rise in pressure. The following fall in the nerve activity occurred at the stage of the second steep rise in pressure. The second increase in the nerve activity was observed after the second steep rise in pressure. The third rise in pressure appeared during the stage of the second increase in sympatheitc nerve activity. The renin release from the kidney increased significantly during the stage of the marked increase in renal sympathetic nerve activity and went up parallel with the stage of the third rise in blood pressure. It is considered that increased renin release from the kidney caused by vertebral artery embolism is due to excitation of the renal sympathetic nerves.

REFERENCES

1. Ueda, H., Yasuda, H. et al.: Increased renin release evoked by mesencephalic stimulation in the dog. Jap. Heart J. 8:498, 1967.
2. Passo, S.S., Assaykeen, T.A., Otsuka, K., Goldfien, A. and Ganong, W.F.: Effect of electrical stimulation of medulla oblongata on peripheral renin activity in dogs. Fed. Proc. 28:579, 1969.
3. Blair, C.S. and Feigl. E.C.: Renin release from brain stimulation. Fed. Proc. 27:629, 1968.
4. Dickinson, C.J. and Yu, R.: Mechanisms involved in the progressive pressor response to very small amounts of angiotensin in conscious rabbits. Circulation Res. 21:157, 1967.
5. Uchida, Y., Ueda, H. et al.: Sympathetic nerve activity during hypertension produced by vertebral embolism. Jap. Heart J. 10: 318, 1969.
6. Ueda, H., Uchida, Y. et al.: Sympathetic activity in cerebral embolism. Jap. Heart J. 10:318, 1969.
7. Helmer, O.M. and Judsen, W.E.: The quantitative determination of renin in the plasma of patients with arterial hypertension. Circulation 27: 1050, 1963.

AREA POSTREMA - ANGIOTENSIN-SENSITIVE SITE IN BRAIN

H. Ueda, S. Katayama and R. Kato

Heart Institute of Japan, Tokyo, Japan and the Second

Department of Internal Medicine, University of Tokyo,

Tokyo, Japan

It is well known that angiotensin has a direct effect on peripheral arterial walls and also acts on brain directly or indirectly
and accordingly elevates the blood pressure. Dickinson and Yu (1)
have demonstrated a pressor response to low concentrations of angiotensin infused into the vertebral artery of rabbits. Similar effects
have been reported in dogs by Scroop and Lowe (2) and in man by Ueda
et al. (3). This study was designed to clarify the central site of
action of angiotensin II by examining the effect of local injection
of angiotensin and the evoked potential of neurons after local and
vertebral artery injection of angiotensin in cats.

A. MICROINJECTION STUDIES

METHODS

Cats(2-3.5 Kg),anesthetized with α-chloralose, were used for
the experiments. Angiotensin II (0.1 to 1.0 µg) dissolved in 3 to
10 µl of artificial cerebrospinal fluid was injected stereotaxically
directly into discrete areas of brain, especially of the brain stem,
of cats through a triple-barrel syringe.

RESULTS

The area which yielded blood pressure responses following
microinjection can be seen on the left of Figure 1. Marked pressor
responses are found mostly at the lateral wall of the fourth ventricle in the medulla, that is, the area postrema. Solid bars in
the right half of Figure 1 represent average pressor responses and

109

the responsive sites are found to be located at the coordinates P_{10} to P_{15}. Microinjection of angiotensin II were also made in 226 points of the upper brain stem as shown in Figure 2. The blood pressure responses are not observed following angiotensin II into these sites.

The pressor response which was obtained when angiotensin was given intramedullarly in a dose of about 1.0 μg as a single injection was almost the same as the response when angiotensin was injected intravenously in a dose 10 to 20 times the intramedullary dose. The nictating membrane contracted more remarkably when angiotensin was injected into the medulla than when it was injected intravenously. These effects are reproducible as shown in Figure 3. Cerebrospinal fluid of the same volume elicited only negligible responses. These results may indicate that the pressor response to microinjection is due to chemical stimulation by angiotensin and not to mechanical stimulation.

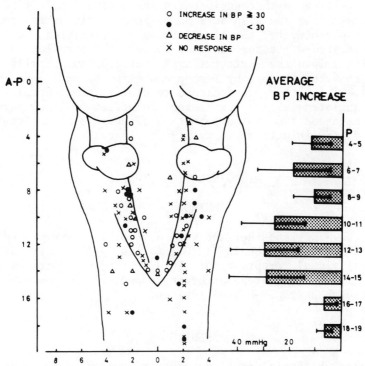

Figure 1.   Localization of blood pressure response to microinjections of angiotensin in cats. Note that the most responsive sites appear to be located at the coordinates P_{10} to P_{15}.

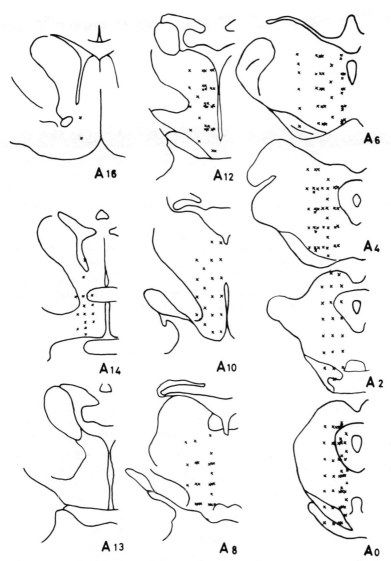

Figure 2. Microinjection of angiotensin into the upper brain stem of cats. No blood pressure response was observed at any of the 226 sites tested.

H. UEDA ET AL.

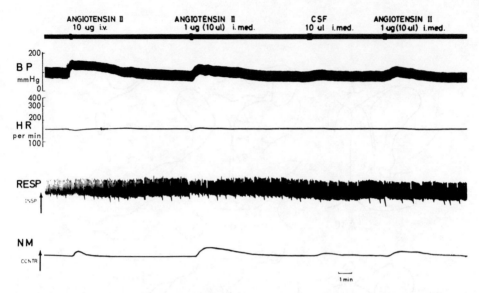

Figure 3.   Effect of angiotensin on blood pressure, heart rate,
            respiration and contraction of the nictating membrane
            in a cat. Note that the nictating membrane contracted
            more markedly after intramedullary injection than
            after intravenous administration.

B. EVOKED POTENTIAL STUDY

METHODS

Cats (α-chloralose anesthetized or immobilized under local anesthesia)were used for the study. The fourth ventricle was exposed and
a tungsten microelectrode was inserted into the area postrema and
other portions of the medulla.   Then, the single discharge of neurons was recorded.   The change of the single discharge was examined
after the microinjection and after vertebral artery injection of
angiotensin II.

RESULTS

The integrated unit activities recorded extracellularly from
the area postrema increased after the vertebral artery injection of
angiotensin as seen in Figure 4.   The unit activities recorded at
the point 2 mm ventral to the former one (Figure 5) showed no
change following vertebral artery injection of angiotensin II.

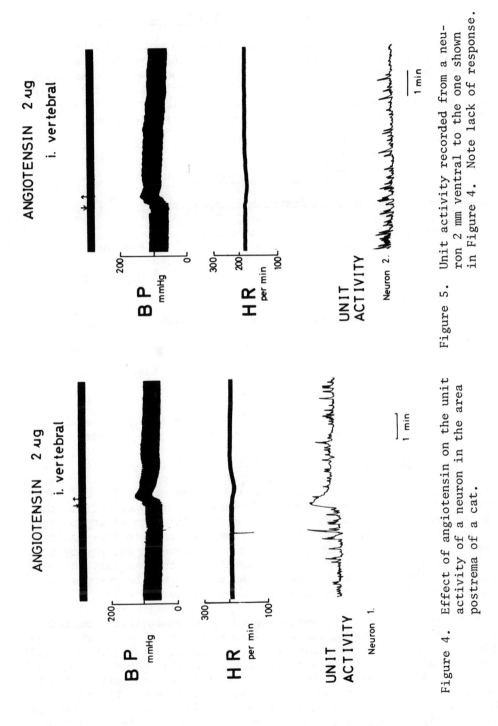

Figure 4. Effect of angiotensin on the unit activity of a neuron in the area postrema of a cat.

Figure 5. Unit activity recorded from a neuron 2 mm ventral to the one shown in Figure 4. Note lack of response.

C. CHEMICAL AND ELECTRICAL STIMULATION OF THE AREA POSTREMA

Electrical stimulation (50 c/s, 2 msec, 3 volts) of the area postrema which is sensitive to angiotensin always produced alterations of blood pressure, chiefly a rise in blood pressure as shown in Table 1. On the other hand, a number of points in the so-called vasomotor area, which are sensitive to electrical stimulation, showed no blood pressure response to chemical stimulation.

TABLE 1

Blood Pressure Response

A. Area Postrema Stimulation

Chemical Stimuli	Electrical Stimuli	
		Pressor 35%
+	+	
		Depressor 9%
+	-	0

B. Vasomotor Area Stimulation

-	+	56%

DISCUSSION

It has been generally recognized that the area postrema is devoid of the blood-brain barrier (4) and angiotensin secretion is found throughout the primates to the lower animals. However, the function of the area postrema is still not clear. Heretofor, the area postrema has been reported to contain the chemoreceptive emetic trigger zone (6) and chemosensitive area to serotonin (7) and catecholamines (8). On the other hand, many authors have noticed the marked pressor response to vertebral artery infusion of angiotensin in low concentrations and have suggested some angiotensin-sensitive area in brain. Therefore, from the pharmacodynamic and phylogenetical point of view, it would be reasonable to suppose that the cell elements near the area postrema in the medulla may be responsible for the mediation of pressor responses to angiotensin II.

We have continued research regarding an angiotensin-sensitive site in the brain during the past five years and have reported preliminary results of these studies on several occasions(8,9,10,11,12). When the author presented a paper on the results ·of microinjection studies last September in Oxford at a meeting of the International Society of Hypertension under the chair of Sir George Pickering, P. Meyer of Paris commented on the relatively high doses of angiotensin II used for microinjection into the area postrema. The effective concentration of angiotensin in dogs was reported as 0.3 to 1.0 ng/ kg/min for 5 minutes (13). We have used 30-500 ng/kg angiotensin dissolved in 3 to 10 µl of artificial cerebrospinal fluid and inject- ed it directly into the area postrema through a triple barrel syringe, stereotaxically. When the area postrema is infused with angiotensin solution via its arterial supply, all the area postrema would be stimulated by angiotensin. On the other hand, very small parts of the area postrema are stimulated with angiotensin by the microinjection method which uses a single injection rather than an infusion. It is not proper to compare the doses of angiotensin used when the routes of administration and the methods of stimulation are different.

A few days after the Oxford Meeting, one of the authors was contacted by investigators at St. Thomas Hospital, London. These investigators showed the author the results of their study (13) on the site of the cardiovascular action of angiotensin II in brain. Their results, using the perfusion method, support our conclusion that the angiotensin-sensitive site in brain is the area postrema. Therefore, the role of the brain stem in the control of the renin- angiotenisn system can be summarized as shown in Figure 6.

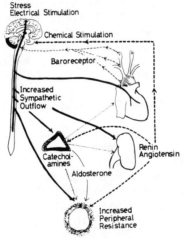

Figure 6.   Schematic view of the relationships between the brain stem and the renin-angiotensin system.

SUMMARY

The site of pressor response on blood pressure in brain to angiotensin II (CIBA) was examined in cats by microinjection of angiotensin II into the brain and by recording the evoked potential after angiotensin administration into the vertebral artery or into the brain directly. It is concluded from the obtained results that the area postrema of medulla oblongata is the site in brain where the angiotensin II reveals pressor effect on blood pressure.

REFERENCES

1. Dickinson, C.J. and Yu R.: Mechanisms involved in the progres-
    sive pressor response to very small amounts of angiotensin in
    conscious rabbits. Circulation Res. 21:157, 1967.
2. Scroop, G.C. and Lowe, R.D.: Central pressor effect of angioten-
    sin mediated by the parasympathetic nervous system. Nature 220:
    1331, 1968.
3. Ueda, H., Uchida, Y. et al.: Centrally mediated vasopressor ef-
    fect of angiotensin II in man. Jap. Heart J. 10:243, 1969.
4. Wislocki, G.B. and Putnam, T.J.: Further observations on the
    anatomy and physiology of the areae postremae. Anatomical Rec.
    27:151, 1924.
5. Wang, S.C. and Borison, H.L.: A new concept of organization of
    the central emetic mechanism: recent studies on the sites of
    action of apomorphine, copper sulfate and cardiac glycosides.
    Gastroenterology 22:1, 1952.
6. Borison, H.L. and Brizzee, K.R.: Morphology of emetic chemore-
    ceptor trigger zone in cat medulla oblongata. Proc. Soc. Exptl.
    Biol. Med. 77:38, 1951.
7. Koella, W.P. and Czicman, J.: Mechanism of EEG synchronizing
    action of serotonin. Am. J. Physiol. 211:926, 1966.
8. Katayama, S., Ueda, H. et al.: Angiotensin and catecholamine
    sensitivity of area postrema. J. Physiol. Soc. Jap. 31:451, 1969.
9. Ueda, H.: Renin-angiotensin system and central nervous system.
    Proceedings of 5th European Congress of Cardiology, pp. 246-252,
    1968.
10. Ueda, H.: Angiotensin-sensitive site in brain. (President's
    speech) J. Jap. Soc. Int. Med. 58:1, 1969.
11. Ueda, H., Katayama, S., et al.: Angiotensin-sensitive neuron in
    medulla oblongata. Jap. J. Med. 9:164, 1970.
12. Ueda, H.: Renin release by catecholamine and angiotensin-sensi-
    tive site in brain stem. Presented at the Meeting of the Inter-
    national Society of Hypertension in Oxford on September 4, 1970.
13. Joy, M.D. and Lowe, R.D.: The site of cardiovascular action of
    angiotensin II in the brain. Clin. Sci. 39:327, 1970.

THE CONTROL OF RENIN RELEASE IN THE NON-FILTERING KIDNEY

J.O. Davis, E.H. Blaine, R.T. Witty, J.A. Johnson,

R.E. Shade, and B. Braverman

Department of Physiology, University of Missouri School

of Medicine, Columbia, Missouri

During the past three years, studies have been conducted on renin release in a non-filtering kidney model in the dog (1-3). The model was developed in order to eliminate the macula densa as an intrarenal receptor. The need for such a model has become increasingly evident in recent years with the failure of experimentation to resolve the major existing problems on the control of renin secretion (4). Most experimental maneuvers which increase renin secretion can conceivably influence both intrarenal receptors, namely, the so-called baroreceptor in the juxtaglomerular cells and the macula densa. Thus, with the non-filtering kidney the functional macula densa was eliminated and dogs prepared in this manner were subjected to hemorrhage or to suprarenal aortic constriction in an attempt to stimulate renal release.

Increased Renin Secretion without Changes in Sodium Delivery to the Macula Densa

The non-filtering kidney model originally was made by clamping both renal arteries for two hours under sterile conditions and by ligating and sectioning both ureters (1). The animals were dialyzed daily for four days and on the fourth day the acute experiment was performed. In conscious dogs, two control samples of blood were obtained from the saphenous vein for measurements of plasma renin activity (PRA) and plasma renin substrate concentration (PRSC) (Figure 1). The dogs were subjected to hemorrhage (20 ml/kg) and peripheral blood samples obtained at 30, 60, and 90 minutes. PRA was increased significantly for all three periods but PRSC was

unchanged. In another group of conscious dogs with non-filtering
kidneys, the animals were subjected to suprarenal aortic constriction as a stimulus for renin release. The response is presented in
Figure 2. Arterial pressure below the constriction was reduced 40-
80 mm Hg. A striking increase in PRA occurred from an average control level of 9.4 nanograms of angiotensin per ml of plasma to 27.3,
33.1 and 37.0 at 30, 60, and 90 minutes respectively; both the 60
and the 90 minute values were highly significant statistically.
Again, PRSC was unchanged. These results show that sodium delivery
to the macula densa was unnecessary for an increase in PRA and, presumably, for increased renin secretion to occur in response to these
two stimuli.

Evidence that these kidneys were non-filtering was provided by
the in vivo visualization of the surface renal tubules through a
dissecting microscope at the end of each individual experiment. To
accomplish this, the dogs were anesthetized after completion of the
experimental procedure and both kidneys were exposed through a long
midline incision. The capsule of each kidney was removed sufficiently to view the surface in three different areas. Lissamine
green dye was injected into the aorta above the renal arteries and
observations made for the passage of dye into surface renal tubules.
The failure of dye to appear in the renal tubules was evidence for
cessation of glomerular filtration.

Two other important lines of evidence were obtained to show
that this model is indeed non-filtering. First, histological sections (1) were made and it was found that the proximal tubules were
filled with casts (Figure 3) so fluid could not be filtered and
flow down the tubules. Second, in a series of 8 dogs (5) the ureter
was reopened and creatinine clearance (C_{Cr}) was measured; the
average value for C_{Cr} was only 2.2 ml/min. This second observation
provides important evidence to demonstrate that even the deep
juxtamedullary nephrons which cannot be evaluated in each individual dog were non-filtering.

Since hemorrhage decreases hepatic blood flow and decreases
the rate of renin metabolism by the liver (6), this mechanism
could conceivably contribute substantially to the increased PRA in
dogs with the non-filtering kidney. However, actual measurements
of the hepatic clearance of renin after a hemorrhage of only 20
ml/kg failed to reveal a detectable decline in renin metabolism
probably because the amount of hemorrhage was too small.

Actual measurements of renin secretion were made to provide
unequivocal evidence that the increase in PRA following hemorrhage
reflected stimulation of the secretory mechanism. For the study
the experimental model and design were changed slightly. The left
renal artery was clamped for two hours under sterile conditions and
the left ureter was ligated and sectioned. Three days later the

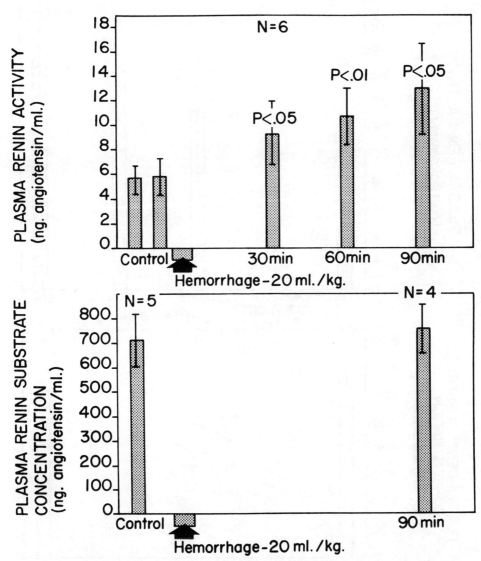

Figure 1.   Response in plasma renin activity to hemorrhage in con-
            scious dogs with non-filtering kidneys.   (Reprinted from
            Circulation Res. 27:1081, 1970 with permission).

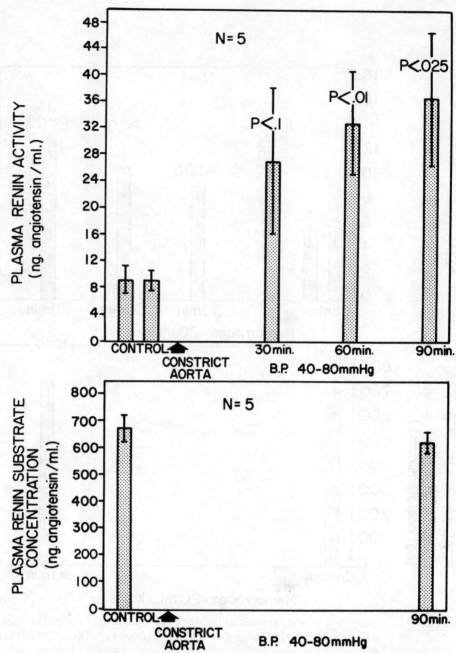

Figure 2.   Response in plasma renin activity to suprarenal aortic
            constriction in conscious dogs with non-filtering kid-
            neys. (Reprinted from Circulation Res. 27:1081, 1970
            with permission.

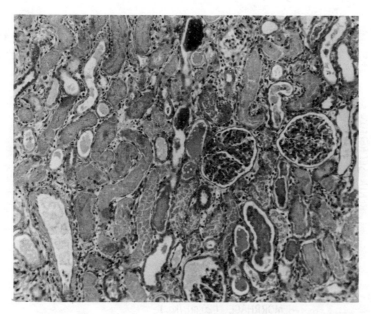

Figure 3.   Photomicrograph of a non-filtering dog kidney which had
             been produced by a 2 hour period of renal ischemia and
             ureteral ligation 4 days earlier (X 125). (Reprinted
             from Circulation Res. 27:1081, 1970 with permission).

right kidney was removed and the following day the acute experiment was performed. The dogs were anesthetized lightly with pentobarbital, renal blood flow was measured with an electromagnetic
flowmeter and the venous-arterial difference of renin across the
kidney was determined. A striking increase in renin secretion
occurred (Figure 4). These data show, therefore, that renin secretion increased following hemorrhage in the absence of changes in
sodium delivery to the macula densa.

Evidence for a Renal Vascular Receptor in
the Control of Renin Secretion

     Since the renal nerves are known to influence renin release,
additional experiments were performed in dogs with denervated, non-
filtering kidneys. Denervation was accomplished at the time of
renal artery clamping and ureteral ligation; the procedure consisted
of removing surgically all nervous connections to the kidney and
applying a 5% phenol solution to the renal vessels. Renal cortical
tissue was analyzed for norepinephrine and the kidneys were found
to be completely denervated since renal cortical norepinephrine was

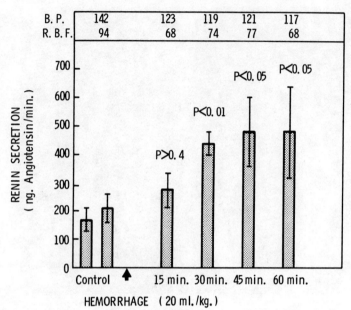

Figure 4. Increased renin secretion by a single non-filtering
           kidney following hemorrhage in dogs (N=5). B.P. and
           R.B.F. are the abbreviations for arterial pressure and
           renal blood flow. (Reprinted from Circulation Res.
           27:1081, 1970 with permission.

almost undetectable by assay. In this experiment, both kidneys
were denervated and non-filtering kidneys made; PRA activity was
measured before and after both hemorrhage and suprarenal aortic
constriction in conscious dogs (Figure 5). A significant increase
in PRA occurred at 30, 60, and 90 minutes after hemorrhage. The
blood was reinfused and the animals were allowed to recover for
three hours before additional observations were made. The second
group of control observations showed that PRA had returned to the
control level. These results demonstrate that hemorrhage with
volume depletion increased PRA while reinfusion of blood and volume
repletion led to return of PRA to the control level. The data are
consistent, therefore, with the existence of a vascular receptor
which responds to changes in vascular volume or possibly to stretch.
An even greater increase in PRA was observed following aortic constriction, a finding also consistent with a stretch or a baroreceptor mechanism since these changes were observed in the non-filtering
kidney. Both the response to hemorrhage and to aortic constriction
occurred without an increase in PRSC. The results suggest that not
only is sodium delivery to the macula densa unnecessary for renin
release but the renal nerves also are not essential.

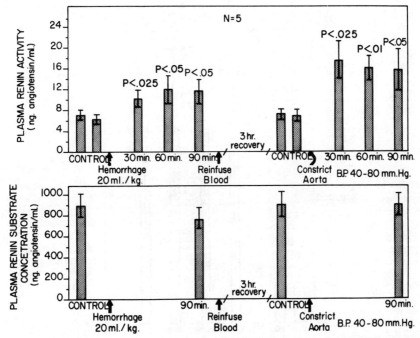

Figure 5.   Changes in plasma renin activity after hemorrhage and
            after suprarenal aortic constriction in dogs with
            denervated, non-filtering kidneys. (Reprinted from the
            Amer. J. Physiol. 220:1593, 1971).

        Finally, because hemorrhage is known to stimulate release of
catecholamines from the adrenal medulla, renin secretion was
studied in the single denervated, non-filtering kidney model in
adrenalectomized dogs. The experimental plan was essentially the
same as in the earlier experiment (Figure 4) except that the left
kidney was denervated and the dogs were adrenalectomized at the
time of surgery to produce the non-filtering kidney. The dogs were
maintained on 50 mg/day of cortisone. In the acute hemorrhage
experiment, renin secretion was significantly increased at 15, 30,
45 and 60 minutes after bleeding (Figure 6). The blood was reinfused in three of the dogs and they were allowed to recover for
two hours. Subsequent suprarenal aortic constriction also increased
renin secretion. In this experiment, it should be emphasized that
increased renin secretion occurred in association with decreased
mean arterial pressure but in the absence of a detectable decline
in renal blood flow. These findings of increased renin secretion
1) in the absence of sodium delivery to the macula densa, 2) by
denervated kidneys, and 3) in the absence of a major portion of
plasma catecholamines in adrenalectomized animals provide strong
evidence for the existence of an intrinsic receptor for renin
release in the renal vascular tree. It should be pointed out,

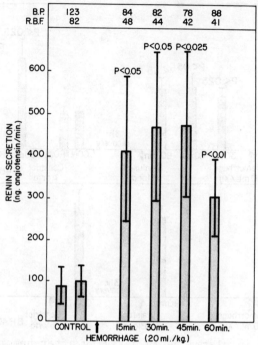

Figure 6.   Increase in renin secretion after hemorrhage in adrenal-
            ectomized dogs with a single non-filtering kidney.
            (Reprinted from the Amer. J. Physiol. 220:1593, 1971).

however, that these observations do not exclude a role for the
macula densa or renal nerves in renin secretion.   Indeed, the fact
that the renin-angiotensin-aldosterone system is so important in
the control of salt and water metabolism makes it likely that more
than one receptor mechanism is operative.

The Effects of Papaverine on Renin Secretion
in the Denervated, Non-Filtering Kidney

        The next experiments were designed to elucidate the nature and
location of the intravascular receptor.   In these studies papaverine
was given into the renal artery in an attempt to dilate the renal
afferent arterioles and to block the increase in renin secretion
which occurs following hemorrhage.   The rationale for this experiment was provided by the observations of Thurau and Kramer (7) who
gave papaverine intrarenally and completely blocked the renal auto-
regulatory mechanism.   Since renal autoregulation is an afferent
arteriolar function, it was reasoned that papaverine might dilate
the renal afferent arterioles and block the response of the vascular
receptor.

Papaverine was infused into the renal artery of dogs with
denervated, non-filtering kidneys. An attempt was made to achieve
maximal arteriolar dilatation with a minimal decrease in arterial
pressure; the average rate of papaverine infusion was 4 mg/min.
While the kidney was receiving papaverine intra-arterially, the
dog was hemorrhaged 20 ml/kg. The response in renin secretion to
hemorrhage was completely blocked (Figure 7). To exclude a possible
toxic effect of papaverine in the blocking of the response in renin
secretion, papaverine was given intrarenally in an identical experiment to dogs with a denervated but filtering kidney (Figure 8). A
highly significant increase in renin secretion occurred in three of
the four periods after hemorrhage. In both groups of dogs, denervation appeared to be complete as revealed by almost undetectable
amounts of renal cortical norepinephrine. Since the block in renin
secretion occurred in dogs with a denervated non-filtering kidney,
the data support our original suggestion that a renal vascular
receptor is involved in renin release. Furthermore, the data are
consistent with an afferent arteriolar locus for the receptor since
papaverine is known to dilate the renal afferent arterioles and to
prevent renal autoregulation.

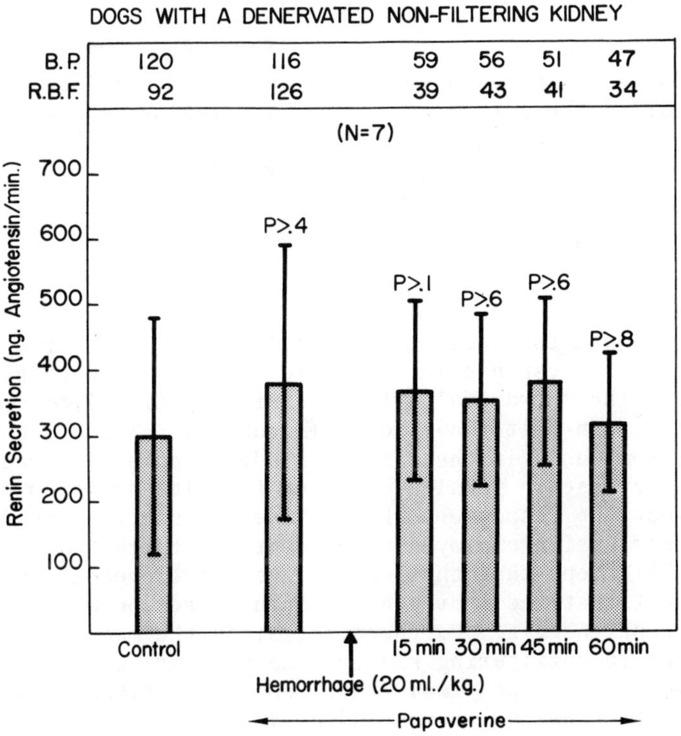

Figure 7. Failure of renin secretion to increase in response to
hemorrhage during the renal intra-arterial infusion of
papaverine with a denervated, non-filtering kidney.
(Reprinted with permission of the Amer. J. Physiol.).

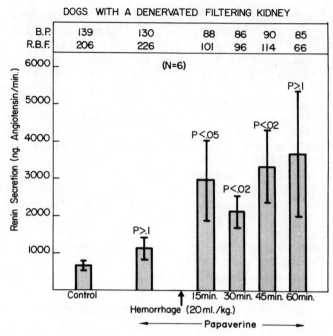

Figure 8.   Increase in renin secretion in response to hemorrhage
            during the intrarenal arterial infusion of papaverine
            into a denervated filtering kidney. (Reprinted with
            permission of the Amer. J. Physiol.).

The Role of the Renal Nerves and Catecholamines
in Renin Release

     To investigate the role of the renal sympathetic nerves in
renin release, the response in renin secretion to hemorrhage was
studied during the intrarenal arterial infusion of papaverine into
the innervated, non-filtering kidney (Figure 9). The design was
identical to that used in the earlier study (Figure 7). Papaverine
produced an increase in renal blood flow from 105 to 143 ml/min but
failed to block the response to hemorrhage. Since the experimental
preparation and design employed were identical to that used earlier (Figure 7) except that the renal nerves were present, the
results suggest that the increase in renin secretion was mediated
through the renal nerves. Furthermore, since the macula densa was
non-functional (non-filtering kidney) and papaverine dilated the
renal arterioles, the data imply that renin secretion was increased
by a direct action of the nerves on the JG cells.

     The next step in these studies of renin secretion in the non-
filtering kidney was to examine the effects of renal nerve stimulation. The renal nerves which lie in close approximation to the

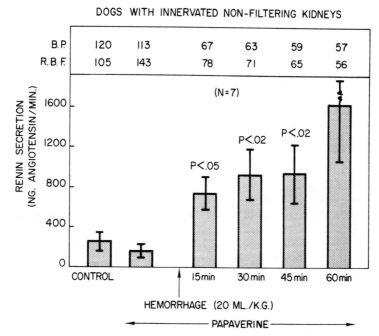

DOGS WITH INNERVATED NON-FILTERING KIDNEYS

B.P.	120	113	67	63	59	57
R.B.F.	105	143	78	71	65	56

Figure 9.   Increase in renin secretion in response to hemorrhage
             during the intrarenal arterial infusion of papaverine
             into an innervated, non-filtering dog kidney. (Reprinted
             with permission of the Amer. J. Physiol.).

renal vessels were stimulated with a Grass model 5 square wave
stimulator with a stimulus duration of 10 msec and a frequency
of 10 pulses per second. The level of voltage used (10-30 volts)
was that necessary to produce a drop in renal blood flow. A
highly significant increase in renin secretion occurred and renin
secretion returned to the control level after cessation of stimulation. In the second part of the experiment, papaverine was infused
intrarenally at a rate to produce a maximal increase in renal blood
flow and the same electrical stimulus applied as before. The
response in renin secretion was almost identical to the increase
observed without the papaverine infusion. The data suggest that
the effects of renal nerve stimulation were mediated by mechanisms
other than 1) the vascular receptor which was presumably blocked
by papaverine, and 2) the macula dense since the response occurred
in a non-filtering kidney. It seems likely that the renal nerves
exerted a direct influence on the JG cells.

     The effects of the intra-arterial infusion of epinephrine and
norepinephrine into the non-filtering kidney before and during the
simultaneous intrarenal infusion of papaverine have also been
studied. Epinephrine alone increased renin secretion but a

concurrent infusion of papaverine completely blocked the response. The dose of epinephrine used (averaged .4 μg/min) was sufficient to decrease renal blood flow slightly less than 50% of the control level; calculations of the renal arterial plasma concentration revealed a level of approximately 11 μg/L. Although this concentration is greater than the basal level of 1 μg/L, it is considerably below the levels of 18-47 μg/L reported (8) during hemorrhage. Since papaverine dilated the renal arterioles and blocked the response to epinephrine, it is suggested that epinephrine exerts an action through the vascular receptor.

Similar studies were carried out with norepinephrine which produced a striking increase in renin secretion in the non-filtering kidney but papaverine failed to block the response. The rate of norepinephrine infused produced a renal plasma level comparable to that observed following acute hemorrhage. These findings suggest, therefore, that in this non-filtering kidney experiment with papaverine the action of norepinephrine was mediated by a direct action on the JG cells. This interpretation is based upon the blocking action of papaverine on the vascular receptor and upon the response occurring in the absence of a functional macula densa. Finally, it should be emphasized that in the normal kidney, a response in renin secretion to the renal nerves, to epinephrine or to norepinephrine may be mediated, at least in part, by way of the macula densa and that the present data do not exclude such a mechanism.

SUMMARY AND CONCLUSIONS

Studies of the non-filtering kidney have provided evidence for an intra-renal receptor in the renal vascular tree which responds to changes in vascular volume and pressure. An intrarenal papaverine infusion completely blocked the response in renin secretion to hemorrhage in the non-filtering kidney, a finding which is consistent with the location of the renal vascular receptor in the renal afferent arterioles. The present observations show that the renal nerves are involved in renin release but are not essential; it is proposed that the renal nerves modulate the control of renin secretion. Epinephrine exerts an action through a non-macula densa mechanism and possibly through a renal vascular receptor; no evidence was obtained for a direct action of epinephrine on the JG cells. Norepinephrine increased renin secretion during papaverine infusion in the non-filtering kidney; these findings suggest a direct action of norepinephrine on the JG cells under these experimental conditions. Finally, the present experiments indicate that the control of renin secretion is regulated by a complex set of mechanisms.

REFERENCES

1. Blaine, E.H., J.O. Davis, and R.T. Witty. Renin release after
    hemorrhage and after suprarenal aortic constriction in dogs
    without sodium delivery to the macula densa. Circulation Res.
    27:1081-1089, 1970.
2. Blaine, E.H., J.O. Davis, and R.L. Prewitt. Evidence for a
    renal vascular receptor in control of renin secretion. Amer.
    J. Physiol. 220:1593-1597, 1971.
3. Blaine, E.H. and J.O. Davis, Evidence for a renal vascular
    mechanism in renin release: new observations with graded
    stimulation by aortic constriction. Circulation Res. 28-29
    (Suppl. II):118-126, 1971.
4. Davis, J.O. What signals the kidney to release renin?
    Circulation Res. 28:301-306, 1971.
5. Johnson, J.A., J.O. Davis, R.E. Shade, and R.T. Witty. Further
    observations on the nonfiltering kidney model: reopening the
    ureter. Fed. Proc. 30:1623, 1971.
6. Johnson, J.A., J.O. Davis, J.S. Baumber, and E.G. Schneider.
    Effects of hemorrhage and chronic sodium depletion on hepatic
    clearance of renin. Amer. J. Physiol. 220:1677-1682, 1971.
7. Thurau, K. and K. Kramer. Weitere Untersuchungen zur myogenen
    Natur der Autoregulation des Nierenkreislaufes. Aufhebung der
    Autoregulation durch muskulotrope Substanzen und druckpassives
    Verhalten des Glomerulus-filtrates. Pflugers Archiv. 269:1,
    77-93, 1959.
7. Manger, W.M., O.S. Steinsland, G.G. Nahas, K.G. Wakim, and
    S. Dufton: Comparison of improved fluorometric methods used
    to quantitate plasma catecholamines. Clin. Chem. 15:1101-
    1123, 1969.

ON THE INTRARENAL ROLE OF THE RENIN ANGIOTENSIN SYSTEM

P. Granger, J.M. Rojo-Ortega, A. Grüner, H. Dahlheim,

K. Thurau, R. Boucher and J. Genest

Clinical Research Institute of Montreal, Montreal,

Quebec, Canada and the Physiological Institute,

University of Munich, Munich, Germany

Several lines of evidence suggest that the function of the renin-angiotensin system is intimately related to renal hemodynamics (1-7), controlling the arteriolo-glomerular balance. The experiments reported here were performed in order to answer the following questions: 1) Is a local formation of angiotensin II in the area of the juxtaglomerular apparatus (JGA) possible ? 2) Do we find contractile structures in the area of the JGA ? 3) Is the renin content of single JGA modified when the distal tubule of the same nephron is perfused with solutions of different sodium concentrations ?

MATERIALS AND METHODS

Renin-Angiotensin-System in Single Microdissected JGA and in the Renal Lymph of Rats

To test the possibility of a local formation of angiotensin II in the area of the JGA the following two experiments were done. First, renin content, converting enzyme and angiotensinase activity were measured in single microdissected JGA of rats. Second, we have measured renin activity, renin substrate and angiotensin I converting enzyme activity in the renal lymph of rats.

Single JGA. Single JGA were microdissected from kidneys in which the vascular tree was injected with Evans blue or Microfil. The glomerulus and the most distal part of the afferent arteriole, equivalent in length to the diameter of the glomerulus together with the tubular tissue in the immediate vicinity of this afferent arteriole were used

for enzymatic determinations. For convenience, these microdissected
structures will be called JGA.

Renin content was measured by the method of Dahlheim and co-
workers (8). In this procedure the availability of a highly purified rat substrate makes possible the determination of the renin content of one JGA within 60 minutes of incubation. Determinations were
done in superficial and juxtamedullary JGA obtained from normal rats
maintained under standard Altromin diet*. The effect of sodium load
and sodium deprivation on renin content of JGA were also studied.
Altromin sodium poor diet was used and sodium rich diet was prepared
by adding 10 gm of NaCl per 100 gm of standard Altromin diet. All
animals were maintained for 30 days under respective diet.

To assay angiotensinase activity of single JGA of normal rats
synthetic valine-5-angiotensin II amide (Hypertensin, Ciba) was used
as substrate. The incubation mixture consisted of 80 ng Hypertensin
per ml of a solution of 150 mM phosphate buffer and 0.1% neomycin
sulfate. Half-life of angiotensin was estimated from a linear plot
on semi-log paper of the exponential disappearance of substrate.

The highly purified renin substrate preparation used for our
determinations of renin content has been previously shown to be devoid of angiotensinase and converting enzyme activity (9). Consequently, a similar incubation mixture as for renin content determination was used for measuring converting enzyme activity of single
JGA of normal rats. Traces of calcium chloride were however added
to the incubation mixture whereas EDTA was not used. Following incubation, the angiotensin formed was measured by rat blood pressure and
rabbit aortic strip assay.

Renal Lymph. To elucidate the possible physiological significance of the renin-angiotensin system in the renal interstitial
space, Horky and Rojo-Ortega (10) in our laboratory have measured
the three main components of this system in the lymph of rat. Lymph
was drained from the lymphatic vessel near to the right renal artery.
The lymph obtained was partly from renal origin since 2 hours following bilateral nephrectomy the lymph flow was significantly reduced
by 38%. Renin activity, renin substrate, and angiotensin I converting enzyme activity (AICEA) were measured by using methods described
by Boucher and co-workers (11,12).

Electron Microscopy of the JGA

In order to give evidence that contractile elements are present
in the area of the JGA, electron microscopic studies of this structure will be presented.

---

* Altromin diet contains 1200 mg sodium / kg diet.

Fixation was done "in-vivo" by injecting the surface of the kidney with 1% osmium tetroxide. Then a small block was cut and post-fixed in the same fixative for one hour. After washing and de-hydration the blocks were included in Epon 812. Thin sections were stained with lead citrate and examined.

Effect of the Distal Tubular Na Concentration on the Renin Content of JGA

Thurau et al. (13) have investigated the influence of various sodium concentrations at the distal tubular site on the renin con-tent of the JGA of the same nephron. Normal rats were prepared as usual for micropuncture. The following experimental procedure was done by two operators with the help of a double stereomicroscope (Figure 1). A 7-μ capillary containing Lissamine Green was used to puncture tubules at random in order to identify proximal and distal segments of a nephron. Then, a 10-μ capillary containing the per-fusion solution was installed in the most superficial proximal seg-ment of the distal tubule. Another capillary with a tip of 15 μ was used to fenestrate the most superficial and distal part of the proximal tubule of the same nephron. Following this fenestration the perfusion of the solution contained in the distal capillary was begun under the control of the two operators. Infusion was made in order to have a retrograde flow escaping through the proximal tubule fenestration. After 10 to 20 minutes of perfusion a fourth capillary

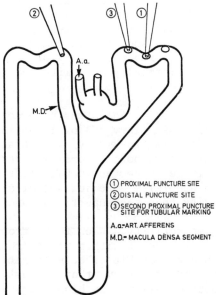

Figure 1.   Experimental procedure for retrograde perfusion of the macula densa segment and marking of the tubule and glomerulus (see text).

containing in its tip Orange Microfil followed by Castor oil was
quickly injected into the proximal tubule, in order to fill the
Bowman's capsule with Microfil. The kidney was then immediately
snap frozen at minus 60° C, removed and freeze dried. This glomerulus with its vascular pole was then microdissected and used for
renin content determination. The glomeruli lying in the vicinity of
the perfused glomerulus were also microdissected and used as controls.
The following solutions were used to perfuse the nephron: 140 mM sodium chloride, 300 mOsm mannitol solution and 260 mOsm choline chloride solution.

RESULTS

Renin-Angiotensin System in Single JGA

Renin Content. Renin content was measured in JGA obtained from
8 rats maintained under Altromin diet. The mean renin content of
superficial and juxtamedullary JGA was essentially the same (Figure
2). A wide scatter was encountered with extreme values from 0 - 42.0.
The values of renin content in JGA obtained from salt loaded and salt
deprived rats are shown in Figure 3. A significant difference was
found when comparing the mean renin content of superficial or juxtamedullary JGA of sodium loaded animals with that of the superficial
or juxtamedullary JGA of salt deprived ones(superf. Na-loaded vs. Na-
deprived: $p < 0.001$; superf. Na-loaded vs. juxtamed. Na-deprived:
$p < 0.01$; juxtamed. Na-loaded vs. superf. Na-deprived: $p < 0.001$;
juxtamed. Na-loaded vs. Na-deprived: $p < 0.001$). The mean renin content of superficial JGA was not statistically different from that of
juxtamedullary ones in both sodium loaded and sodium deprived rats.
In sodium restricted rats, renin activity of superficial JGA was
slightly higher but statistically not different from that of juxtamedullary JGA.

Angiotensinase Activity. Angiotensinase activity was determined
in superficial and juxtamedullary JGA of 13 normal rats. Results are
illustrated in Table 1. In two kidneys (no. 6 and 13) angiotensinase
activity was undetectable in both superficial and juxtamedullary JGA.
In another kidney a longer Hypertensin half-life was associated with
juxtamedullary JGA. Otherwise the juxtamedullary JGA had a higher
angiotensinase activity than the superficial ones.

Converting Enzyme Activity. When renin from a single microdissected JGA was allowed to react with purified renin substrate the
angiotensin formed had comparable effects on rat blood pressure and
rabbit aortic strip. Table 2 shows that in most of the cases the
effects of the incubation mixture on blood pressure and rabbit aortic
strip were similar. When the same purified rat renin substrate was
incubated with purified rat renin*, conversion of less than 15% was
obtained.
_____
* Generously donated by Dr. Haas, Cleveland.

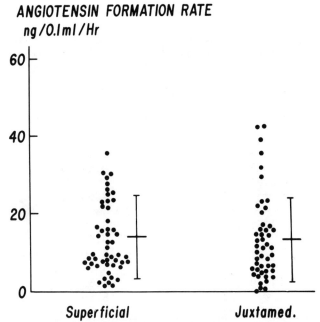

Figure 2.   Renin activity of superficial and juxtamedullary JGA
of rats maintained under standard Altromin diet.

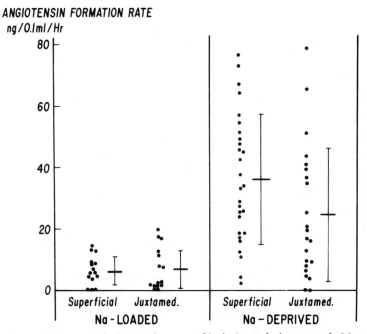

Figure 3.   Renin activity of superficial and juxtamedullary JGA
of sodium-deprived and sodium-loaded rats.

TABLE 1

Half-Life (Hour) of Added Synthetic Valine 5 Angiotensin II Amide with Single Superficial and Juxtamedullary JGA of Rats.

	JGA	
	Superficial	Juxtamedullary
1	12.48 (5)	8.83 (5)
2	4.18 (4)	3.61 (4)
3	13.25 (4)	10.50 (4)
4	5.68 (4)	
5	∞ (6)	7.90 (5)
6	∞ (4)	∞ (5)
7	4.55 (5)	5.49 (6)
8	∞ (5)	9.60 (6)
9	7.80 (5)	5.80 (5)
10	9.10 (5)	3.17 (5)
11	14.10 (6)	2.35 (5)
12	∞ (6)	5.50 (6)
13	∞ (6)	∞ (6)

Figures in brackets give the number of determinations.

TABLE 2

Identification of the Angiotensin* Formed by
Single JGA After 1 Hour of Incubation (ng/0.1ml/h)

Rat Blood Pressure		Rabbit Aortic Strip	
30	11	60	13
20	14	< 6	12
7	11	< 6	13
26	15	26	12
29	20	29	58
11	13	< 6	6
13	9	14	10
15	8	< 6	14
8	14	< 6	8

* Rat blood pressure and rabbit aortic strip assays
were used to differentiate angiotensin I from II.

Renin Activity, Renin Substrate and AICEA
in the Renal Lymph of Rats.

The studies on the three main components of the renin angiotensin system in the renal lymph of rats showed the following results
(Table 3). Renin, renin substrate and angiotensin I converting enzyme activity were all present in the renal lymph. Moreover, 2 hours
following bilateral nephrectomy renin and AICEA were found to be
decreased in both plasma and lymph.

TABLE 3

Renin Activity, Renin Substrate and Angiotensin I
Converting Enzyme in the Lymph and in the Left
Renal Venous Plasma of Rats.

	Lymph	Renal Venous Plasma
Renin Substrate ng/ml/hr	35.1 ± 6.7	34.2 ± 4.3
Renin Activity ng/ml/hr	4.1 ± 0.4	8.9 ± 1.6
AICEA ng/hr	395.0 ±61.6	426.0 ±73.7

* Mean followed by ± standard error.

Electron Microscopy of the JGA

Myofilaments are present in a) smooth muscle cells and endothelial cells of both afferent and efferent arterioles, b) granular
epitheloid cells and c) mesangial cells.

However, renin producing cells always have myofilaments and in
many occasions dense attachment bodies. Figure 4 shows these structures in an epitheloid cell.

Effect of the Distal Tubular Na Concentration
on the Renin Content of JGA.

Retrograde mannitol perfusion of distal tubule and Henle's loop
was done in 12 nephrons (Table 4). Renin content in perfused JGA
was slightly lower than in control JGA. Following perfusion with
choline chloride solution in 9 nephrons, renin content in perfused

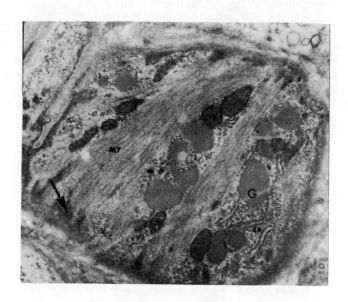

Figure 4.   Electron micrograph (magnification: 25,000) of a granular epitheloid cell. My: Myofilament. G: Granule. E.R.: Rough endoplasmic reticulum. Arrow shows dense attachment body.

TABLE 4

Renin Activity (ng/0.1ml/h) of Single JGA's
Mannitol Perfusion (300 mosm/L)

| Exp.No. | CONTROL | | | | PERFUSION |
	Single Values			Mean	VALUE
1	2.4	1.0	1.3	1.6	1.4
2	18.6	19.6	15.8	18.0	21.6
3	24.4	17.7	49.7	30.6	27.7
4	37.0	13.8	32.4	27.7	8.4
5	12.1	9.9	23.8	15.3	17.8
6	27.7	20.6	23.4	23.9	21.1
7	17.0	19.0	14.5	17.1	10.3
8	6.0	11.0	13.0	10.0	9.6
9	13.2	14.2	33.0	20.1	9.5
10	30.0	40.0	41.2	37.1	2.8
11	17.0	28.4	5.0	16.8	8.6
12	12.2	5.5		8.8	8.0
			Mean (SD)	18.9 ± 9.9	12.2 ± 8.0

TABLE 5

Renin Activity (ng/0.1ml/hr) of Single JGA's
Choline Chloride Perfusion (265 mosm/L)

| Exp.No. | CONTROL | | | | PERFUSION VALUE |
	Single Values			Mean	
1	15.2	21.0	12.0	16.1	12.0
2	28.5	55.5	43.5	41.5	15.3
3	7.1	7.6	7.9	7.5	5.8
4	7.3	7.7	6.6	7.2	7.9
5	12.6	11.1	13.7	12.5	11.4
6	12.7	12.9	11.3	12.3	12.0
7	10.0	7.0	9.6	8.9	10.0
8	1.1	10.5	4.4	5.3	2.4
9	8.0	13.0	21.0	14.0	15.0
			Mean (SD)	13.9 ± 10.9	10.2 ± 4.2

TABLE 6

Renin Activity (ng/0.1ml/hr) of Single JGA's
Sodium Chloride Perfusion ([Na] = 140 mEq/L)

| Exp.No. | CONTROL | | | | Mean | PERFUSION VALUE |
	Single Values					
1	5.8	5.7	3.2	6.3	5.3	13.8
2	27.0	8.7	7.1	27.0	17.5	34.0
3	34.4	28.2	14.0	33.2	27.5	66.0
4	22.4	22.0	8.8		17.7	42.0
5	5.8	16.8	10.8		11.1	32.1
6	9.6	3.2	19.0		10.6	16.0
7	20.8	12.0	9.6		14.1	28.0
8	25.6	13.6	8.6		15.9	26.0
9	19.2	4.8	15.6		13.2	21.6
10	18.3	22.3	24.1		21.6	47.2
11	5.4	25.2	12.7		14.4	45.4
12	2.8	1.6			2.2	18.0
13	2.1	9.9			6.0	30.9
14	9.4	10.5			9.9	78.8
			Mean (SD)		13.4 ± 6.7	35.7 ± 18.8

JGA was not different from control ones (Table 5). Fourteen nephrons were perfused with 140 mM (Table 6) sodium chloride. Renin
content in these perfused JGA (35.7) was significantly higher than
in control ones (13.4) ($p < 0.001$).

DISCUSSION

Renin Angiotensin System in JGA and in the
Renal Lymph of Rats

Previous studies have shown that renin is located in the granular cells of the afferent arteriole (14-21). We have provided additional evidence for the presence of renin in the JGA. However,
we failed to find a different renin content between juxtamedullary
and superficial JGA of normal rats. Sodium restriction and sodium
loading respectively increased or decreased renin content of both
superficial and juxtamedullary JGA. In sodium restricted rats mean
renin content of superficial JGA was slightly higher but statistically not different from that of juxtamedullary JGA.

The discrepancies between our results and those of Gavras and
co-workers (22) are most probably due to species difference. We
have obtained preliminary results indicating that there is in rab-
rits' kidneys a much higher renin activity in superficial JGA than
in juxtamedullary ones.

Our results of similar renin content in superficial and juxtamedullary JGA are also at variance with the measurement of juxtaglomerular index (JGI) in superficial and juxtmedullary JGA. It is
established that juxtamedullary JGA in the rat have a lower JGI (23).
Such a dissociation between JGA renin and JGI between superficial
and juxtamedullary JGA is however observed by Brown and co-workers
(24) following renal artery constriction in the rabbit. We have
also observed in newborn dogs despite the absence of granules in the
afferent arteriole a normal renin content in renal cortex and a very
high plasma renin compared to the normal adult dog (25).

Angiotensinase activity was shown to be higher in juxtamedullary
JGA. This activity could be associated with structural components of
the glomerular tuft or the vascular pole. It is known that juxtamedullary glomeruli are larger than the superficial ones in rats (26)
and this difference in size could explain the higher activity.

Our results for converting enzyme activity in single microdissected JGA were supported by the observation of angiotensin converting enzyme activity in the renal lymph of rat. Moreover renin activity and renin-substrate were also found to be present in the lymph.
The presence of renin and its substrate in renal lymph of dogs was
reported by Lever and Peart (27) and by Hosie et al. (28). Different

workers gave evidence that part of the angiotensin I passing through the kidney was converted to angiotensin II (29-32).

The local formation of angiotensin II in the area of the JGA seems possible since renin, renin substrate, converting enzyme activity and angiotensinase activity are all present in this area.

Electron Microscopy of the JGA

The renin producing cells always have myofilaments and in many occasions dense attachment bodies are observed. Therefore, it would be possible that part of the arteriolar resistance at that level could be due to the contraction of the granular epitheloid cells of the afferent arteriole in response to local formation of angiotensin II. This suggestion does not exclude the possibility that the locally formed angiotensin II could act on other contractile structures of the arteriolo-glomerular complex since myofilaments are also present in the smooth muscle cells and endothelial cells of afferent and efferent glomerular arterioles, and in the mesangial cells.

Effect of the Distal Tubular Na Concentration on the Renin Content of JGA

The group of Thurau (5,6) reported micropuncture experiments which indicated that the JGA controls the filtration rate and hence the tubular sodium load of its own glomerulus. Recently Schnermann et al. (7) provided direct evidence that in superficial nephron the glomerular filtration rate was related to the amount of sodium delivered to the distal tubule. To evaluate the possibility that a variable, local, formation of angiotensin II was involved in such a feedback mechanism, the content of renin of single JGA was measured following retrograde perfusion of its macula densa segment with solutions of different sodium concentration and compared to non-perfused JGA obtained from the same kidney. Renin content was higher in JGA following perfusion of their macula densa segment with 140 mM sodium chloride solution. This was not the case when iso-osmotic mannitol or choline chloride was perfused. These data are consistent with the hypothesis that the renin angiotensin system in single nephron is involved in a tubulo-vascular feedback mechanism.

CONCLUSION

The effective angiotensin level present at the site of the JGA may not be predicted from measurements of renin activity in these JGA. The angiotensinase activity varies from superficial to juxtamedullary JGA. We have also obtained results which are consistent

with the presence of converting enzyme activity in the area of the
JGA. There exists evidence that renin substrate is certainly available in the surroundings of the JGA since it is present in renal
lymph. These factors are all involved in the turnover of angiotensin and its direct determination is required to prove definitely a
control of glomerular filtration mediated by the renin-angiotensin
system.

The data presented, however, suggest that the enzymes required
for a local formation of angiotensin II in the JGA are present in
this area. The epitheloid cells of the afferent arteriole as well
as the smooth muscle cell from this arteriole contain contractile
structures which render possible a local action of angiotensin II.

As one possible mechanism of control of single nephron filtration rate by the sodium in the macula densa tubular fluid, a local,
variable formation rate of angiotensin II in the area of the JGA was
considered. In order to test this hypothesis the content of renin
in the vascular pole of single rat glomeruli was determined after
their macula densa segment had been retrogradely perfused with sodium chloride solution at 140 mM. The data obtained are consistent
with a physiological function of the renin angiotensin system in an
intrarenal feedback control of single nephron filtration rate by
tubular sodium chloride concentration at the level of the macula
densa.

REFERENCES

1. Goormaghtigh, N.,Les segments neuro-myoarteriels juxtaglomerulair-
   es du rein. Arch. Biol. 43:575, 1932.
2. Goormaghtigh, N.,Facts in favor of an endocrine function of the
   renal arterioles. J. Path. Bact. 57:392, 1932.
3. Guyton, A.C., Langston, J.B., Navar, G.,Theory of renal autoregulation by feedback at the juxtaglomerular apparatus. Circulation
   Res. 14: Suppl. I, 187, 1964.
4 Vander, A.J., Miller, R.,Control of renin secretion in the anesthetized dog. Am. J. Physiol. 207:537, 1964.
5. Thurau, K., Schnermann, J.,Die Natriumkonzentration an den Macula
   Densa-Zellen als regulierender Faktor für das Glomerulumfiltrat.
   Klin. Wochschft. 43:410, 1965.
6 Thurau, K. Proc.,3rd Intern. Congress Nephrol. ed. by Schreiner,
   G.E., Washington, D.C., Vol. 1, 162, 1966. S. Karger.
7. Schnermann, J., Wright, F.S., Davis, J.M., Stackelberg, W., Grill,
   G.,Regulation of superficial nephron filtration rate by tubulo-
   glomerular feedback. Pflügers Arch. 318:147, 1970.
8. Dahlheim, H., Granger, P., Thurau, K.,A sensitive method for determination of renin activity in the single juxtaglomerular apparatus
   of the rat kidney. Pflügers Arch. 321:303, 1970.

9. Thurau, K., Dahlheim, H., Granger, P., On the local formation
   of angiotensin at the site of the juxtaglomerular apparatus.
   Proc. 4th Intern. Congress Nephrol., Stockholm 1969, Vol. 2,
   p.24. S. Karger.

10. Horky, K., Rojo-Ortega, J.M., Rodriguez, J., Boucher, R. and
    Genest, J., Renin, renin substrate, and angiotensin I convert-
    ing enzyme activity in the lymph of rats. Am. J. Physiol. 220:
    307, 1971.

11. Boucher, R., Menard, J., Genest, J., A micromethod for measure-
    ment of renin in the plasma and kidney of rats. Can. J. Physiol.
    Pharmacol. 45:881, 1967.

12. Boucher, R., Kurihara, H., Grise, C., Genest, J., Measurement
    of plasma angiotensin I converting enzyme activity. Circulation
    Res. 27: Suppl. I, 83, 1970.

13. Thurau, K., Dahlheim, H., Grüner, A., Mason, J., Granger, P.,
    The dependence of renin activity in the single juxtaglomerular
    apparatus of the rat nephron upon NaCl in the fluid of the macula
    densa segment. Intern. Congress Physiol. Sci., Munich, 1971.

14. Bing, J., Wiberg, B., Localization of renin in the kidney. Acta
    Pathol. Microbiol. Scand. 44:138, 1958.

15. Cook, W.F., Pickering, G.W., The location of renin in the rabbit
    kidney. J. Physiol. 149:526, 1959.

16. Bing, J., Kazimierczak, J., Localization of renin in the kidney
    II. Acta. Pathol. Microbiol. Scand. 47:105, 1959.

17. Bing, J., Kazimierczak, J., Further studies on the localization
    of renin in the kidney. Ann. Histochem. 6:537, 1961.

18. Bing, J., Kazimierczak, J., Renin content of different parts of
    the juxtaglomerular apparatus. 4. Localization of renin in the
    kidney. Acta Pathol. Microbiol. Scand. 54:80, 1962.

19. Bing, J., Eskildsen, P.C., Faarup, P., Frederiksen, O., Location
    of renin in kidneys and extrarenal tissues. Circulation Res. 20:
    Suppl. II, 21, 1967.

20. Brown, J.J., Davies, D.L., Lever, A.F., Parker, R.A., Robertson,
    J.I.S., Assay of renin in single glomeruli. Lancet 2:668, 1963.

21. Cook, W.F., The detection of renin in juxtaglomerular cells. J.
    Physiol., London 194:73, 1968.

22. Gavras, H., Brown, J.J., Lever, A.F., Robertson, J.I.S., Changes
    of renin in individual glomeruli in response to variations of
    sodium intake. Clin. Sci. 38:409, 1970.

23. Rojo-Ortega, J.M., Genest, J., Index de l'activite histochimique
    de la glucose-6-phosphate dehydrogenase dans la macula densa et
    sa distribution dans le cortex renal chez le rat. Path. Biol.18:
    595, 1970.

24. Brown, J.J., Davies, D.L., Lever, A.F., Parker, R.A., Robertson,
    J.I.S., The assay of renin in single glomeruli and the appear-
    ance of the juxtaglomerular apparatus in the rabbit following
    renal artery constriction. Clin. Sci. 30:223, 1966.

25. Granger, P., Rojo-Ortega, J.M., Perez, S., Boucher, R., Genest,
    J., The renin angiotensin system in newborn dogs. Canad. J.
    Physiol. Pharmacol. 49:134, 1971.

26. Baines, A.D., de Rouffignac, C., Functional heterogeneity of
    nephrons. II. Filtration rates, intraluminal flow velocities
    and fractional water reabsorption. Pflügers Arch.308:260,1969.
27. Lever, A.F., Peart, W.S., Renin and angiotensin-like activity
    in renal lymph. J. Physiol. 160:548, 1962.
28. Hosie, K.F., Brown, J.J., Harper, A.M., Lever, A.F., MacAdam,
    R.F., MacGregor, J., Robertson, J.I.S., The release of renin
    into the renal circulation of the anesthetized dog. Clin. Sci.
    38:157, 1970.
29. Gocke, D.J., Gerten, J., Sherwood, L.M., Laragh, J.H., Physiol-
    ogical and pathological variations of plasma angiotensin II in
    man: correlation with renin activity and sodium balance. Circu-
    lation Res. 24: Suppl. I, 131, 1969.
30. Oparil, S., Sanders, C.A., Haber, E., In-vivo and in-vitro con-
    version of angiotensin I to angiotensin II in dog blood. Circu-
    lation Res. 26:591, 1970.
31. Franklin, W.G., Peach, M.J., Gilmore, J.P., Evidence for the
    renal conversion of angiotensin I in the dog. Circulation Res.
    27:321, 1970.
32. Bailie, M.D., Rector, F.C., Seldin, D.W., Angiotensin II in
    arterial and renal-venous plasma and renal lymph in the dog.
    J. Clin. Invest. 50:119, 1971.

RENIN RELEASE BY RAT KIDNEY SLICES IN VITRO

M.H. Weinberger and D.R. Rosner

Renal-Hypertension Laboratory, Department of Medicine,

Indiana University School of Medicine, Indianapolis,

Indiana

The stimuli for renin release have been a source of considerable interest as evidenced by the work of the past several years and the communications of this conference. Today I would like to describe a method whereby isolated stimuli can be examined for their effect on renin release from rat kidney slices in vitro. This method has been developed and refined in our laboratory and we are currently beginning studies to elucidate the factors that control renin release in vitro.

Table I outlines briefly the method that we have developed. We use rats of the Wistar strain (200 ± 25 gm) and, except for special studies that I will present shortly, utilize regular laboratory chow as diet. Under barbiturate anesthesia (Nembutal, 50-60 mg/kg) bilateral nephrectomy is performed by paravertebral incisions. Four, 10-20 mg slices are prepared from each kidney using a Stadie-Riggs microtome. Each slice is pre-incubated for 15 minutes in a beaker containing 2.0 ml of Robinson's media (1) in a shaking incubator at 25°C with 95% O_2-5% CO_2 saturated atmosphere. We have found oxygen consumption to be lower and renin release longer at 25°C than at 37°C. The control media has been modified to an osmolal concentration of 350 mOsm/L by the addition of mannitol. The pre-incubation media is aspirated and the slice is incubated with 2.0 ml fresh media (control or experimental) for 30 minutes as described above.

We add 0.1 ml renin-containing media from the kidney slice incubate to 0.4 ml of our current substrate preparation and incubate for 3 hours at 37°C in a shaking incubator. The angiotensin I thus generated is quantitated by the radio-immunoassay technique of Haber and colleagues (2) and expressed as ng/mg dry kidney weight. Substrate is prepared from the plasma of 48 hour post-nephrectomy dogs

TABLE I

Study of Renin Release by <u>In Vitro</u> Rat Kidney Slices

1. Wistar rats (200 ± 25 gm)

2. Barbiturate anesthesia (Nembutal)

3. Nephrectomy - prepare 10-20 mg slices (dry) (4 slices/
   kidney - Stadie-Riggs microtome)

4. Pre-incubation of slice X 15 minutes in 2.0 ml Robinson's
   media at 25°C, shaking incubator with 95% O_2 - 5% CO_2

5. Aspiration of pre-incubation media and incubation with
   fresh media (experimental or control) X 30 minutes as in #4

6. Incubation of 0.1 ml renin-containing media with 0.5 ml
   substrate at 37°C X 3 hours in shaking incubator

7. Quantitation of angiotensin I generated by radio-immunoassay
   (Haber et al.)

collected in 2.6 mM EDTA, by a differential ammonium sulfate pre-
cipitation (3) and stored at 4°C until used.

Table 2 demonstrates the effect of increasing substrate concentration on angiotensin I generation. Both media and substrate
contain 2.6 mM EDTA, 1.6 mM BAL and 3.4 mM 8-OH quinoline to inhibit
converting enzyme and angiotensinase activity. We have taken
optimal substrate concentration as 0.4 ml of our present preparation
per 0.1 ml of renin-containing media. Substrate incubated alone
and renin-containing media alone generated negligible amounts of
angiotensin I.

Early in our studies we examined the effect of variation in
sodium chloride concentration on renin release. At the time of
these experiments the media used was Kreb's Ringer bicarbonate,
containing sodium bicarbonate rather than balanced sodium and
potassium phosphate as buffers in Robinson's media. We used substrate prepared from the plasma of nephrectomized rats at that time.
From these studies indicated in Table 3, optimal sodium concentration appears to be between 119 and 238 mM. To assess the effect of
a low sodium diet on the rats prior to preparation of the kidney
slices, we performed the study summarized in Table 4. Paired
slices from rats fed a low sodium diet for the indicated time were
incubated with control Kreb's media (119 mM) or with media to which
NaCl had been added (1190 mM). The high sodium media appeared to
reduce renin release to a similar level in each group studied.

TABLE 2

Effect of Increasing Substrate Concentration on
Angiotensin I Generation

Renin-containing media	Substrate	Angiotensin I (ng/ml/45 min)
0.1 ml	0.1 ml	321
0.1 ml	0.2 ml	439
0.1 ml	0.3 ml	428
0.1 ml	0.4 ml	402
0.1 ml	0.5 ml	344
-	0.4 ml	0.07
0.8 ml	-	0.36

TABLE 3

Effect of Sodium Concentration on Renin Release
(Kreb's Bicarbonate Media-Nephrectomized Rat Substrate)

Sodium Concentration	(n)	Angiotensin I (ng/mg dry kidney) ± SD
11.9 mM	(16)	606 ± 71
119 mM	(47)	1180 ± 132
238 mM	(8)	1210 ± 241
595 mM	(8)	786 ± 34
1190 mM	(16)	312 ± 28

TABLE 4

Effect of Low Dietary Sodium Intake on Renin Release by Rat Kidney
Slices (Angiotensin I Generation ng/mg ± SD)

Days of Diet	119 mM NaCl	1190 mM NaCl	(p)
2	735.5 ± 162	264.5 ± 19.3	< 0.05
5	1350 ± 395	349.8 ± 101	0.05
6	2687 ± 608	408 ± 105	< 0.01
combined	1698 ± 256	342.9 ± 47.1	< 0.001

However, the amount of renin release by the kidney slice pair
incubated in control media increased with the duration of the low
sodium diet.   It has been shown (4) that renin release in vitro is
related to renal renin content.   These studies suggest that renal
renin content increased during sodium deprivation.

After the modifications in our procedure that led to the method
that I just described, namely the use of substrate prepared from
nephrectomized dog plasma and the use of Robinson's media, we
evaluated whether the previous effect of variation in NaCl concentration could be mediated by changes in the osmolality of the media.
The osmolality of the media was increased from the control level of
350 mOsm/L, by the addition of choline chloride, to 550, 750 and
950 mOsm/L.   Table 5 depicts the results obtained from comparing
renin release by one of a pair of slices incubated at successively
increasing osmolal concentrations, with the other slice of the pair
kept at 350 mOsm/L.   The osmolal optimum appears to be 550 mOsm/L,
similar to the osmolality of the optimum sodium chloride concentration (238 mM) in Table 3.

The last experiment, summarized in Table 6 indicates the observations made when sodium chloride concentration was varied, but the
osmolality of the media kept constant at 550 by the addition (or
deletion) of choline chloride.   There is no significant difference
through a 7-fold range of sodium chloride concentration in this
experiment.

In summary, we have developed a sensitive method of studying
renin release by isolated stimuli in the rat kidney slice in vitro.
It would appear from the studies reported here, that the effect of
variations in sodium chloride concentration, in this isolated system, are mediated by changes in osmolality.   We are currently util-
izing this technique to further study stimuli affecting renin re-

TABLE 5

Effect of Osmolality on Renin Release in Rat Kidney Slices
(Robinson's media-nephrectomized dog substrate)

media osmolality (mOsm/L)	% of control angiotensin generation (ng/mg)
350	100 ± 22
550	149 ± 26
750	130 ± 27
950	139 ± 29

(n = 8 paired slices)

TABLE 6

Effect of Variation in [NaCl] on Renin Release in Rat Kidney Slices
(Robinson's media + choline chloride/NaCl to constant 550 mOsm/L)

[NaCl] (mM)	% of control angiotensin I generation (ng/mg) ± SD
237.5	97.1 ± 28.3
187.5	107.9 ± 36.7
87.5	97.5 ± 33.6
37.5	101.5 ± 35.5

(n = 12 paired slices)

lease in vitro. We have recently received confirmation of the increased efficiency of the 25°C incubation temperature and the osmolal effect of variations in sodium chloride concentration from
studies performed independently by Dr. K. Yamamoto and colleagues
in Osaka, Japan (5).

REFERENCES

1. Robinson, J.R., Biochem. J. 45:68, 1949.
2. Haber, E., Koerner, T., Page, L.B., Kliman, B. and A. Purnode, J. Clin. Endocr. 29:1349, 1969.
3. Skeggs, L.T., Lentz, K.E., Hochstrasses, H. and J.R. Kahn, J. Exp. Med. 118:73, 1963.
4. Braverman, B., Freeman, R.H. and H.H. Rostorfer, Proc. Soc. Exp. Biol. Med. 134:67, 1970.
5. Yamamoto, K., personal communication.

CONVERSION OF ANGIOTENSIN I TO II IN VIVO AND IN VITRO

S. Oparil and E. Haber

Cardiac Unit, Medical Services, Massachusetts General

Hospital and the Department of Medicine, Harvard Medical

School, Boston, Massachusetts

It has long been believed that the conversion of the inactive decapeptide hormone angiotensin I (AI) to angiotensin II (AII) was mediated by a plasma dicarboxypeptidase (1). More recently the provocative experiments of Ng and Vane (2) suggested that the major site of conversion was the pulmonary circulation and that conversion in plasma could not account for the rapid pressor response to an intravenous injection of AI.

In order to define more precisely the site and specificity of the conversion reaction both in plasma and in the intact animal, detailed studies employing synthetic labeled peptides (3) and peptides with altered sequence (4) were undertaken. The techniques of radiochromatography and radioimmunoassay (5,6) were used to identify and quantify reaction products.

Conversion in Plasma and Blood

The rates of conversion of AI to AII were studied in plasma treated with several anticoagulants as well as in whole blood. The study of conversion is complicated by the simultaneous degradation of AII as indicated in Figure 1. Two methods were used for study of conversion rates. In one approach, the release of labeled products was measured. Asp^1-Ile^5 ^3H-$Leu^{10}AI$ was incubated with blood or plasma and products identified by high voltage paper electrophoresis, and quantified by liquid scintillation counting. Conversion rates were determined by decrease in AI radioactivity. In the second method the release of AII from unlabeled AI was determined by specific radioimmunoassay for AII. Table 1 shows the

152   S. OPARIL AND E. HABER

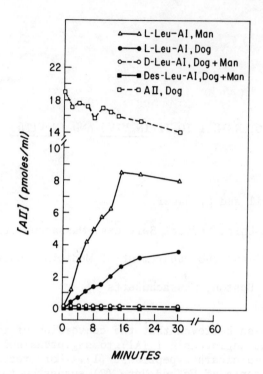

Figure 1.   In vitro metabolism - diluted plasma. The level of
            AII activity is plotted against time. Starting con-
            centration of each peptide was 20 pmoles/ml. (Repro-
            duced from Reference #4)

TABLE 1

Half Time for Conversion (min)*

Medium	Persistence of ^{3}H AI	Radioimmunoassay of AII
Plasma - Heparin	10	------
Plasma - Citrate	30	------
Plasma - EDTA	240	------
Whole Blood (without anticoagulation)	3	10

*Half times for conversion were arrived at by extrapolation from
at least 4 experiments under each condition.

half times for conversion in undiluted plasma and whole blood. It
is clear that the presence of anticoagulants retards conversion.
Under optimal circumstances, in non-anticoagulated whole blood, the

half time for conversion as determined by persistence of ^{3}H AI was three minutes. This would tend to underestimate conversion times, because AI is simultaneously attacked by both converting enzyme and other proteases. The 10-minute half time for AII release in whole blood tends to overestimate conversion times since AII is also rapidly degraded under these circumstances. If the correct half time lies between 3 and 10 minutes, it cannot account for the rapid pressor response seen in one circulation time after intravenous injection of AI.

Figure 2 shows the products of plasma conversion with the various anticoagulants employed. The first product is clearly His-Leu. His-Leu also appears first on incubation of AI in whole blood, though more rapidly. Apparently His-Leu is later degraded to component amino acids, since the final product on prolonged incubation is ^{3}H Leu.

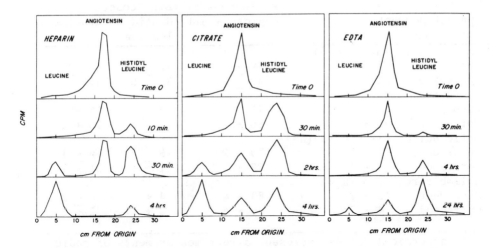

Figure 2.   Angiotensin I conversion, dog plasma in vitro. Paper electrophoresis strips of plasma samples anticoagulated with heparin, citrate, and EDTA and incubated with ^{3}HAI for the specified periods of time. The positions at which standards migrated are labeled at time 0. Radioactivity is quantified as counts per minute (CPM). Each initial ^{3}HAI peak contained approximately 5,000 CPM. (Reproduced from Reference #3)

In order to examine the specificity of plasma converting enzyme, two analogs of AI [D-Leu^{10}AI and Des-Leu^{10}AI] were synthesized by the solid phase technique. Figure 1 shows that in diluted plasma conversion to AII can be readily demonstrated for L-Leu AI, whereas D-Leu AI or Des-Leu AI release no AII.

Conversion In Vivo

Conversion in vivo in the intact dog was examined by injection of peptides into the pulmonary artery or right ventricle and collection of samples from the aorta. Products were analyzed either by radiochromatography or radioimmunoassay as indicated previously. Central arterial pressures were simultaneously monitored. Table 2 indicates that 53+3% of injected AI was converted to AII in a single passage through the pulmonary circulation as determined from measurement of radioactively labeled peptides.

TABLE 2

Angiotensin I Conversion in Vivo in Intact Dogs

Apparent percent conversion		Percent of total counts		
		Angiotensin I	Histidyl leucine	Leucine
Pulmonary circulation(n=5)				
Uncorrected	61 + 3	39 + 3	14 + 4	47 + 7
Corrected	53 + 3	47 + 3	11 + 5	42 + 7
Renal circulation(n+4)				
Uncorrected	24 + 2	76 + 4	8 + 1	16 + 2
Corrected	20 + 2	80 + 4	7 + 1	13 + 2
Hepatic portal circulation(n=4)				
Uncorrected	22 + 3	79 + 9	15 + 2	6 + 1
Corrected	2 + 1	98 + 9	1 + 1	1 + 1
Hindlimb circulation(n=4)				
Uncorrected	12 + 2	88 + 4	4 + 1	8 + 2
Corrected	4 + 2	96 + 4	2 + 1	2 + 1

The uncorrected values represent direct measurements of radioactively labeled peptides. The corrected value is arrived at by subtracting the percent conversion which would occur in dog blood at 37° in a comparable period of time. The mean value + 1 SE is given for each experimental group. (Reproduced from Ref. #3).

These data were confirmed by radioimmunoassay measurements which showed 54% release of AI under similar circumstances (Table 3). A pressor response occurred within 15 seconds. Since a single circulation in this preparation is 15 seconds, conversion in the

lung is clearly more rapid than in plasma or whole blood as discussed previously.

TABLE 3

Angiotensin I Conversion Measured by Radioimmunoassay

	Angiotensin I		Angiotensin II	
	μμmoles/ml	Percent	μμmoles/ml	Percent
Pulmonary circulation(n=2)	192-212	46	275-300	54
Renal circulation				
High dose(n=4)	98-555	93 ± 1	7-29	7 ± 2
Low dose(n=8)	41-100	91 ± 2	5-13	9 ± 1

The quantities of angiotensin I and II are expressed as μμmoles/
ml plasma and as percents of total immunoreactive activity in each
sample. The range of absolute values and the mean percent ± 1 SE
are given for each experimental group. (Reproduced from Ref. #3)

Similar studies were carried out in other organs, injecting
peptide into the renal artery, hepatic portal vein, and femoral
artery and sampling from the renal vein, hepatic vein and femoral
vein respectively. Table 2 summarizes the results of these experiments. It is apparent that the kidney is the only organ other
than the lung which shows evidence for conversion. These observations were also confirmed by measurement of AII in the renal venous
effluent by radioimmunoassay.

The major product of conversion in the lungs and kidneys
appeared to be ^{3}H Leu. However, ^{3}H His-Leu was 50% degraded to
^{3}H Leu in a single circulation time in the lungs. It was, consequently, not clear whether Leu was a primary product of pulmonary
converting enzyme or a secondary product of His-Leu degradation.

In order to determine whether pulmonary converting enzyme
acted as a mono or dicarboxypeptidase, D-Leu AI and Des-Leu AI
were injected into the pulmonary artery of dogs and the aortic
samples analyzed after a single circulation by radioimmunoassay.
The results are summarized in Table 4. It is apparent that neither
of these peptides is converted to AII. AI, under these circumstances, results in a prompt pressor response; no pressor response
is seen with the other peptides.

TABLE 4
Pulmonary Conversion - in Vivo

Peptide Injected	Concentration in Arterial Blood			
	Injected Peptide		Angiotensin II	
	pmoles/ml	percent	pmoles/ml	percent
L-Leu-AI (n=6)	17.3±3.4	44.1±4.0	22.4±2.7	56.2±7.3
D-Leu-AI (n=6)	33.6±2.8	96.4±1.5	1.25±0.5	3.6±0.4
Des-Leu-AI (n=6)	Not Measurable		0.9±0.2*	-
Control (no peptide injected)	0.1±.05		0.05±0.02	

* This number does not differ significantly from that accounted for
by cross reactivity with estimated venous concentration of Des-Leu
AI.   The mean value ± 1 SE is given for each experimental group.

DISCUSSION

Angiotensin I is converted to angiotensin II in the pulmonary
circulation at a more rapid rate than can be demonstrated in unal-
tered blood. The capacity of the lung for conversion is sufficiently great so that at 10,000-fold the physiologic concentration
of AI, 50% conversion can be demonstrated in a single circulation
time. The renal circulation also appears to participate in conversion, but its capacity is less. The mechanism of action and
specificity of the enzymes at the two sites appears to be similar.
Plasma converting enzyme has previously been shown to be a dicarboxypeptidase (1). This was confirmed by demonstrating the inability
of this enzyme to convert Des-Leu AI to AII. In vivo, Des-Leu
AI is also not converted to AII in the pulmonary circuit, nor does
it result in a pressor response. It is likely, then, that ^{3}H Leu
demonstrated in vivo as the major product of AI conversion was the
result of secondary degradation of His-Leu in the pulmonary circulation. It is of interest that dipeptidase action is for more
rapid in the lungs than in plasma or blood (3). The inability of
either plasma or pulmonary converting enzyme to attack D-Leu AI
indicates the importance of the structure of the carboxyl terminus
in determining the specificity of the converting enzymes.

ACKNOWLEDGEMENTS

The research presented was supported by USPHS Grants HE-14150,
HE-44850, HE-5196 and NASA Grant NGR 22-016-0007.

REFERENCES

1. Skeggs, L.J., Kahn, J.R., and Shumway, N.P.: Preparation and function of the hypertension-converting enzyme. J. Exp. Med. 103:295, 1956.
2. Ng, K.K.F., and Vane, J.R.: Conversion of angiotensin I to angiotensin II. Nature(London) 216:762, 1967.
3. Oparil, S., Sanders, C.A., and Haber, E.: In-vivo and in-vitro conversion of angiotensin I to angiotensin II in dog blood. Circulation Res. 26:591, 1970.
4. Oparil, S., Tregear, G.W., Koerner, T., Barnes, B.A., and Haber, E.: Mechanism of pulmonary conversion of angiotensin I to angiotensin II in the dog. In press. Circulation Res.
5. Haber, E., Koerner, T., Page, L.B., Kliman, B., and Purnode, A.: Application of a radioimmunoassay for angiotensin I to the physiologic measurements of plasma renin activity in normal human subjects: renin activity by angiotensin I radioimmunoassay. J. Clin. Endocr. 29:1349, 1969.
6. Page, L.B., Haber, E., Kimura, A.Y., and Purnode, A.: Studies with the radioimmunoassay for angiotensin II and its application to measurement of renin activity. J. Clin. Endocr. 29:200, 1969.

RENAL MEDULLARY MECHANISMS RELATING TO HYPERTENSION

L. Tobian, Jr. and S. Azar

Department of Medicine, University of Minnesota

Minneapolis, Minnesota

Since this is a renin workshop, I would like to report one study involving renin. We produced a form of experimental hypertension by feeding 8 % NaCl to rats for 7 weeks followed by 7 weeks of feeding ordinary Purina chow. Some rats remained hypertensive after 7 weeks on a normal salt intake and they are said to have "post-salt" hypertension. One possible reason for this hypertension is the development of arterial and arteriolar lesions during the period of high salt intake. Such a state of affairs should be accompanied either by normal or high levels of plasma renin. It would also be possible that other mechanisms play a part and they might conceivably bring about a low level of circulating renin. To investigate this problem, we quickly obtained arterial blood from 23 rats with "post-salt" hypertension (BP 180-240) and from 21 normotensive control rats (BP 113-135). Renin levels were determined with the Boucher method. The plasma of the hypertensive rats averaged 188 ng/10ml/3hr of "renin units". The plasma of the normotensive control rats averaged 174 "renin units". This difference was definitely not significant with the t value of the difference being 0.3.

This result does not disavow the concept that the permanent hypertension is the consequence of lesions narrowing the afferent arterioles in the kidney. It would be compatible with such a hypothesis. Of course, it certainly does not rule out other causes of the permanent hypertension. Now to discuss another subject.

Over the past two years, we have been looking at the interstitial cells of the renal papilla in relation to high blood pressure. Figure 1 shows a diagram of one of these cells which appear abundantly in the kidney of man, rat and rabbit. They lie horizontally in the interstitial spaces between loops of Henle, capillaries and collecting ducts. They are especially unique in that they have many

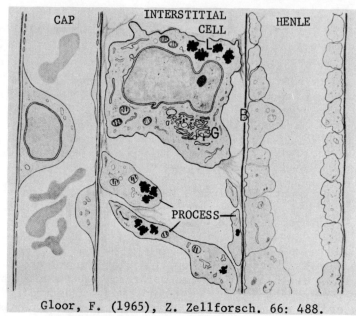

Gloor, F. (1965), Z. Zellforsch. 66: 488.

Figure 1.   A diagram of an interstitial cell in the renal papilla
            (after Gloor).   The black spots are the cytoplasmic
            lipid granules.

cytoplasmic granules filled with a lipid material.   These cells appear to have some secretory function, which probably involves the
secretion of a lipid substance.   Figure 2 is an electron micrograph
of one of these cells.   The black blobs in the figure are the lipid-
filled osmiophilic granules.

One can also see these granules by light microscopy.   In Figure
3 the section on the right is from a normal rat renal papilla and
one can see many black dots which represent the lipid granules in
the interstitial cells.   The section on the left is from the renal
papilla of a hypertensive rat.   In three different types of rat
hypertension and even in severe human hypertension, there is a definite scarcity of interstitial cell granules.

Lipid substances extracted from the renal medulla can lower the
blood pressure of hypertensive animals.   Renal transplantation in
man convinces us that the normal kidney somehow exerts an anti-
hypertensive action.   Lipid agents coming from the renal medulla
could be involved in this anti-hypertensive effect.   The obvious cell
to carry out such a function would be the highly specialized interstitial cell with its many lipid granules.   Moreover, the scarcity
of lipid granules in hypertensive rats might mean that these cells

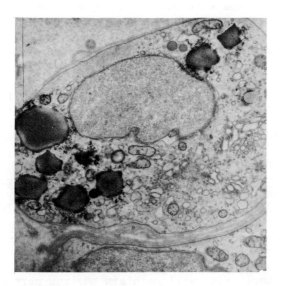

Figure 2. An electron photomicrograph of an interstitial cell.
The black blobs are the lipid granules.

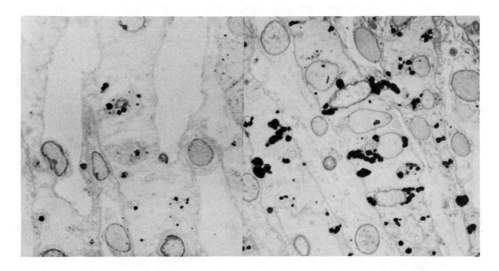

Figure 3. Photomicrographs of the renal papilla stained with
methylene blue-azure II. The frame on the right is
from a normal rat and has many black dots representing
the many lipid granules in the interstitial cells. The
frame on the left is from a rat with "post-salt" hypertension. It shows a paucity of lipid granules.

had become atrophic and were no longer capable of secreting an anti-hypertensive substance. This would be roughly analogous to the atrophic, degranulated beta cells in the pancreatic islets in severe juvenile diabetes. To test this proposition, we set up two separate types of experiments.

In the first experiment, we recognized that the papilla of the kidney secretes a large amount of prostaglandin E_2. The granules of the interstitial cells contain triglyceride with an unusually large amount of arachidonic acid, which is the biochemical precursor of prostaglandin E_2. It seemed highly likely that the E prostaglandins are secreted by these specialized interstitial cells. Such prostaglandin could even act as an anti-hypertensive hormone. We thus undertook to measure the release of E prostaglandin by the renal papilla as an index of the secretory activity of the interstitial cells. We were comparing papillas from rats with "post-salt" hypertension versus papillas from normotensive control rats. The rats with "post-salt" hypertension were fed a diet with 8 % sodium chloride for 7 weeks and then fed ordinary Purina chow for an ensuing 5 weeks. Some of these rats will maintain their hypertension indefinitely while eating regular chow and thus have "post-salt" hypertension. In each comparison we would quickly obtain a renal papilla from each of 6 hypertensive rats and cut it longitudinally in half. The resulting 12 papilla halves were put into an oxygenated medium similar to a Krebs-glucose-bicarbonate solution except that the sodium and urea concentrations were raised, and the oxygen tension was lowered to resemble conditions in the renal papilla. Twelve papilla halves from 6 normotensive control rats were placed at the same time into another similar flask. Both flasks were gently shaken for exactly two hours at 37° C and then the bathing medium from each flask was subjected to a series of solvent extractions to isolate the acidic lipids. This fraction was then run on a thin layer chromatograph. The spot that corresponds to prostaglandin E_2 was then eluted and bioassayed on a colonic muscle strip.

Eight comparisons of this type were done. Each line in Figure 4 represents one comparison, with the normal papillas on the left side of Figure 4 and the hypertensive papillas on the right side. Each dot gives the nanograms of E prostaglandin secreted into the medium per 180 mg of papilla. In seven out of eight comparisons, the hypertensive papillas released more prostaglandin than the normal papillas. Averaging all the comparisons, the hypertensive papillas put out 56 % more prostaglandin than the normal papillas, with a p value of 0.01.

The next test of this hypothesis involved Muirhead's method for implanting fragments of renal medulla. In Muirhead's experiments, these implanted fragments release humoral agents which have an anti-hypertensive action. Our recipient animals were rats with "post-salt" hypertension. Their blood pressure was taken every other day

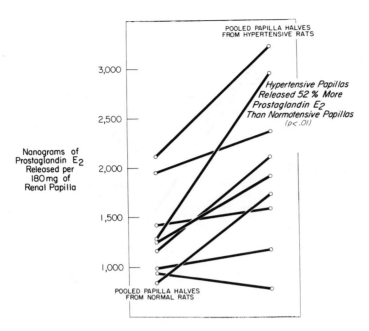

Figure 4.   Eight comparisons of hypertensive and normotensive
            papillas in regard to their release of prostaglandin
            E_2 into a modified Krebs-Henseleit medium.

until five readings were obtained. The average of these five readings was considered the initial blood pressure. These hypertensive
rats were then divided into three groups as shown in Figure 5. The
23 hypertensive rats represented by the middle line of Figure 5 received fragments of normal renal papilla by subcutaneous injection.
Each rat received 0.4 gm of these fragments.

     Each of the eight hypertensive rats in the group represented
by the bottom line of Figure 5 also received papillary fragments,
but in this case the fragments were obtained from the kidneys of
rats with "post-salt" hypertension.

     Each of the 15 hypertensive rats represented by the top line
of Figure 5 received only a subcutaneous injection of the diluent
solution. The blood pressure of all rats was carefully measured on
the fourth day after papillary implantation, since rejection of the
implants would be expected to increase substantially after this time.
The average initial blood pressure was about the same for all three
groups and way above the normal average of 130. The injection of
the diluent alone lowered the pressure an average of 8 mm Hg. In
the 23 rats that received implants of normal papillas, the blood
pressure fell an average of 23 mm Hg. This drop was significantly
greater than that with diluent alone.

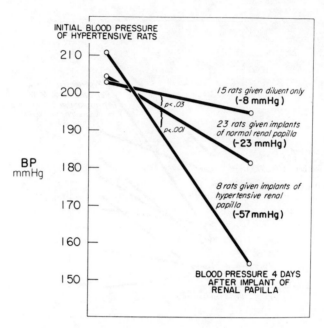

Figure 5.   The lowering of blood pressure in hypertensive rats
             after the subcutaneous implantation of fragments of
             renal papilla.

And in the 8 rats that received the implant of hypertensive
papilla, the blood pressure fell an average of 57 mm Hg. This fall
in pressure was significantly greater than that seen with implants of
normal papilla.

Many typical interstitial cells have been seen in these medullary implants. We can thus confirm Muirhead's observation that
implanted fragments of normal renal medulla have an anti-hypertensive
action. Moreover, implanted fragments from hypertensive renal medulla have an even greater anti-hypertensive effect. These studies indicate that hypertensive papillas are quite capable of secreting
anti-hypertensive agents and prostaglandins and are therefore not
comparable to the atrophied beta cells in severe juvenile diabetes.
Thus, the rat with "post-salt" hypertension is not hypertensive because of an utter inability of the renal papilla to secrete prostaglandins and other anti-hypertensive materials.

It is intriguing that the separated papillas of hypertensive
rats actually secrete more prostaglandin and have more anti-hypertensive action than normal. At least two broad speculations come
to mind. First, it is possible that the intact papilla in the hypertensive rat is actually secreting large amounts of anti-hypertensive
material in vivo in an attempt to bring the blood pressure down, but

such a valiant effort is of no avail. A second possibility is that
the conditions of blood pressure or blood flow or fluid composition
or hormonal substances in the hypertensive kidney influence the
interstitial cells to hold their anti-hypertensive materials in ab-
eyance. Then when the papilla is removed from these influences and
put into quite a different environment, as in our experiments, it
may commence to secrete anti-hypertensive agents at a rapid rate.
We need much more information to unravel this problem.

In a third study involving the interstitial cells, we gave rats
all their calories as a dilute drinking fluid for 2 weeks. Such rats
undergo a brisk water diuresis since they drink a daily volume of
fluid equal to 3/4 of their body weight. Two groups of rats were
compared: one group drinking all calories as a dilute suspension
containing 38 % of calories from safflower oil; the other group
drinking all calories as a dilute suspension with 38 % of calories
from butter fat. In this study, we also had 11 rats eating regular
dry chow and water ad libitum. As seen in Table 1, the average interstitial cell granule count in this normal control group was 147.
The 12 rats drinking the fluid containing butter fat had an average
granule count of 85, a marked reduction below the control value. The
12 rats drinking the fluid containing safflower oil had an average
granule count of 158, a value actually slightly higher than that in
the control group. Obviously, the rats on butter fat had a marked
reduction in granules compared to the rats on safflower oil and the
difference was highly significant. This study indicates that the

TABLE 1

Interstitial Cell Granule Counts in Normal Rats and
in Rats Undergoing Water Diuresis

	Papillary Interstitial Cell Granules (average granule count)
11 normal control rats eating dry chow and water ad lib	147
12 diuretic rats with butter fat as 38 % of calories	85
12 diuretic rats with safflower oil as 38 % of calories	158

The p value of the difference between the two
diuretic groups is less than 0.0001.

number of granules can be strikingly dependent on the polyunsaturated
or saturated fatty acids in the diet. One could speculate that the
forced water drinking stimulates hypersecretion by the interstitial
cells. If the E prostaglandins were hypersecreted, they would further diminish the effect of the low level of ADH that might be present and thus facilitate maximum water diuresis. This hypersecretion
would use up precursor materials in the granules, especially arachidonic acid which is needed for the synthesis of E_2 prostaglandins.
A diet stressing butter fat provides only a limited amount of polyunsaturated fatty acids. This would retard the replenishment of
polyunsaturated lipid in the granules and thus lead to a sharp drop
in the number of granules. With a diet stressing safflower oil,
there is a great abundance of polyunsaturated fatty acid. This
would permit the granules to be replenished with polyunsaturated
lipid, thus preventing a drop in the granule count. At any rate,
during water diuresis, the number of granules is remarkably dependent on the availability of polyunsaturated fatty acids.

THE ROLE OF THE RENIN-ANGIOTENSIN SYSTEM IN CONTROL OF ALDOSTERONE SECRETION

J.R. Blair-West, J.P. Coghlan, D.A. Denton, J.W. Funder,

and B.A. Scoggins

Howard Florey Institute of Experimental Physiology and

Medicine, University of Melbourne, Parkville, Australia

The discovery in 1953 by the Taits and colleagues of the electrolyte active hormone aldosterone was a major landmark in the understanding of sodium homeostasis (1). Soon after, Bartter, Mills, Biglieri and Delea showed an influence of blood volume change on rate of aldosterone secretion (2). Laragh and Stoerk found increase of K intake increased aldosterone secretion (3). Several groups of investigators demonstrated that the anterior pituitary had an important but restricted role in the control of secretion in different species. The successful implementation of the idea of autotransplanting the left adrenal gland with attached renal vessels to a combined carotid artery-jugular vein skin loop in the neck of the Merino sheep, giving free access to artery and venous drainage in the conscious animal (4,5), was followed by demonstration that physiological decrease in plasma [Na] or increase in [K] acted directly on the adrenal to stimulate aldosterone secretion (6,7). The small rate of blood flow through the adrenal made it possible to produce locally in adrenal blood a wide range of change in composition with negligible systemic effect of the infusion. Thus it was possible formally to define precisely those factors which acted directly on the adrenal and those factors which, though influential on adrenal secretion, acted via an intermediate vector.

An early finding with this preparation was that increasing arterial plasma [Na] to normal level or above in the Na deficient animal had only a small effect on the aldosterone hypersecretion, and thus plasma [Na] change was not a major factor in the response to Na deficiency (6). In 1958, Denton, Goding and Wright reported

discovery of an unidentified aldosterone stimulating hormone by
cross circulation experiments on conscious sheep (6). A Na deficient adrenalectomized animal was donor and the blood was led to
the adrenal transplant of a Na replete recipient. Concurrently
and independently, Yankopoulis, Davis, Kliman and Peterson reported
the same result in the anaesthetized dog, the donor having the
thoracic vena cava constricted (8). In the light of recent data
presently to be described, the development of emerging experimental
ideas at this time is of particular interest.

In 1958 we suggested (6) that "alternative to the usual view
that the adrenal controlled the kidney in certain respects, the
kidney might be the site of a receptor sensitive to haemodynamic
change or supply of Na, and accordingly secrete an adrenotrophic
hormone", and that the receptor mechanism, whether in the same
place as the tissue secreting the hormone or not, is - "(a) akin
to a Na accounting machine, in that, for example, serially arranged
transfer mechanisms in a specific local vascular field register the
load of Na/unit time in the local blood supply; or that (b) volume
change causes stimulation of a pressure or stretch receptor or
determines the area of surface available for particular transfer
process". These proposals are not unlike some facets of current
views of the pathway of aldosterone control through renin (9).
However, we found Na deficiency caused increased aldosterone secretion in the nephrectomized animal - a finding ostensibly against a
renal control of aldosterone. Retrospectively, in the face of data
strongly in favour of renal control, we wholly attributed this
earlier result to ionic effects. This may now have to be re-
evaluated in the light of evidence of new factors in aldosterone
control. Davis, in view of our result with nephrectomy, first
examined the effect of hepatectomy on aldosterone hypersecretion in
response to haemorrhage, found the response unchanged, and then
made the important finding that nephrectomy did abolish this
response (10). Ganong and Mulrow independently reported the same
result (11). Gross in 1958 made the inspired suggestion, on the
grounds of inverse relation between sodium balance on the one hand
and renin content of kidneys and aldosterone on the other, that the
renin system may play an important role in aldosterone secretion (12).
This discovery of a major role of the kidney in aldosterone hypersecretion was followed by the demonstration by Genest's (13) and
Laragh's (14) groups that intravenous infusion of angiotensin II
stimulated aldosterone. Our laboratory showed that the action of
angiotensin II was directly upon the adrenal transplant and not via
a secondary pathway (7). It was shown that nephrectomy reduced
aldosterone hypersecretion of Na deficiency to basal in dog (15)
and sheep (16). With the development of the enzyme kinetic assay
for renin, and the radioimmunoassay for angiotensin II, it was shown
by groups at St. Marys London (17), the College of Physicians New
York (18) and ourselves (19) that renin and angiotensin are increased

in Na deficiency. Angiotensin II has been widely accredited with the dominent role in physiological control of aldosterone secretion, as stated in 1965 by Binnion et al (20), - "increased activity of the renin-angiotensin system is the primary mechanism leading to hyperaldosteronism during Na depletion."

In this paper, we wish to present a re-appraisal of this view set against some long standing doubts we have expressed, and new evidence of the existence of an unidentified humoral factor(s) in aldosterone control. That is, in the absence of changes in the other known factors in aldosterone control - i.e., plasma [Na], [K] and ACTH. - the rate of secretion of aldosterone is not simply and directly determined by the contemporary level of angiotensin II in the blood. The role of angiotensin II is important in secondary hyper-aldosteronism, but may be restricted to a permissive or a contributory causal role in concert with another factor/factors, which remain to be identified.

In sheep with adrenal auto-transplants, onset and development of Na deficiency can be contrived by continuous uncompensated loss of saliva from a permanent parotid fistula. Aldosterone secretion, blood angiotensin II concentration and plasma renin concentration rise commensurately with Na deficit (19). All four factors are highly significantly correlated - a strong prima facie case for primacy of the renin-angiotensin system in the light of the known action of angiotensin on aldosterone secretion (21). A similar finding has been made in man (18). However, the following series of findings from experiments in sheep are not easily reconciled with a simple and direct control of aldosterone in Na deficiency by angiotensin II. Clear-cut dislocation of the usual parallel change of angiotensin II and aldosterone levels in Na deficiency has been contrived with some procedures.

1. Angiotensin II infusion, intravenous or adrenal arterial, does not increase aldosterone secretion in moderately sodium deficient sheep (22,23) whereas increase of Na deficiency does (Fig. 1). If the moderate rate of aldosterone secretion represented the mid range of an angiotensin aldosterone dose-response curve, the increased angiotensin II level would consistently elevate the aldosterone secretion commensurately with infusion rate. Adrenal arterial K infusion increases aldosterone secretion in the moderately Na deficient sheep (19).

2. Continuous intravenous or adrenal arterial infusion of angiotensin II, or intravenous infusion of sheep renin does not sustain a high aldosterone secretion rate beyond 6-12 hours in sodium replete sheep, though the pressor action is maintained (7.19). This transient effect may be a consequence of the frequent concurrent hypokalaemic alkalosis induced by the intravenous angiotensin infusion. The result with adrenal arterial infusion remains (Fig.2 and 12) unexplained on this basis.

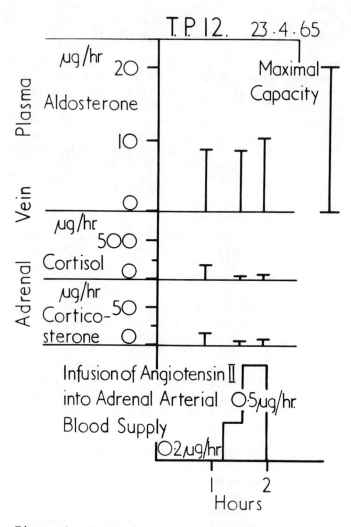

Figure 1. Transplant 12 - Mild-moderate Na deficiency. Adrenal arterial infusion of angiotensin II at 0.2 - 0.5 µg/hr, a rate which has an aldosterone stimulating effect in the Na replete animals, **did not increase aldosterone** secretion. The panel on the right shows the rate of aldosterone secretion observed in this animal with severe Na deficiency.

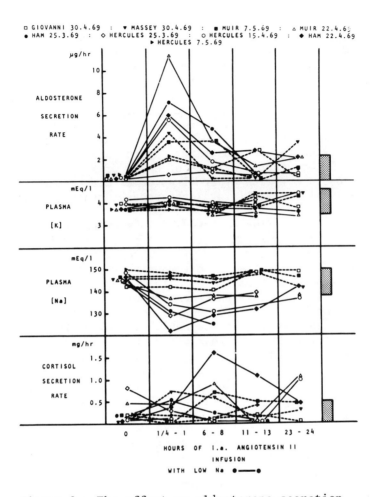

Figure 2. The effect on aldosterone secretion
of adrenal arterial infusion of angiotensin II
over 24 hours at rates calculated to give adrenal
blood concentrations of angiotensin II equivalent
to those observed in peripheral blood in Na deficiency. In one group of experiments (● ------- ●)
the sheep were given infusion of angiotensin II in
isotonic saline, in another group (● _____ ●)
antiogensin II was infused in 5% mannitol so that
plasma [Na] was decreased concurrently with increase
of blood angiotensin II concentration. The effect
on aldosterone secretion was not maintained in
either instance.

3. The in-vivo biosynthesis of aldosterone has been studied
by adrenal arterial infusion of radiolabelled corticosterone. With
the onset and development up to the middle range of aldosterone
response to Na deficit, an increased percentage conversion of ^{3}H-
corticosterone to ^{3}H-aldosterone was observed. With severe Na
deficit the percentage conversion fell again to the Na replete
range. This change in the biosynthetic process, as Na deficiency
progressed, indicated a two-component system (19,24,25). When
aldosterone secretion was stimulated acutely over comparable range
by concurrent adrenal arterial infusion of angiotensin II, the rapid
rise of aldosterone was not associated with increased per cent conversion of corticosterone substrate. Angiotensin II infusion did
not mimic the biosynthetic effects of onset of Na deficiency. The
finding is consistent with other lines of evidence of an early site
of action of angiotensin II in aldosterone biosynthesis (26).

4. Sheep were sodium depleted by loss of parotid saliva for
2-3 days, and then permitted to rapidly correct deficiency by
drinking 2-3 L of hypertonic $NaHCO_3$ solution (300 mEq/L) over 5-15
minutes. By two hours later aldosterone secretion rate was substantially dissociated from angiotensin II level. A mean aldosterone
fall of over 50% occurred without change of mean blood angiotensin
II concentration (27). By 4-6 hours aldosterone secretion was
basal, whereas angiotensin II and renin levels remained in the moderately Na deficient range. This effect was associated with ionic
changes. However, if the same range of plasma ionic changes,
increased [Na], [HCO_3] and pH, and decreased [K], were produced
locally by adrenal arterial infusion of hypertonic $NaHCO_3$, the fall
of aldosterone secretion was significantly less (28).

5. This quantitatively suggestive result, though not
conclusive, led to design of experiments in which large variation
of Na status was contrived under conditions where blood angiotensin
II was held relatively invariant throughout the experiment. In a
large series of experiments, a constant infusion of angiotensin II
amide was given at either 10, 20, 60, or 100 µg/hr for four days.
The resultant blood levels covered the range seen in mild to very
severe Na deficiency (10 - 100 ng/100 ml). The animals were kept
Na replete for the first 24 hours of angiotensin II infusion, and
then allowed to become depleted of 500 - 900 mEq of Na as a result
of salivary loss over two days. Finally they were permitted to
correct Na deficiency by rapidly drinking 2-3 L of $NaHCO_3$
(300 mEq/L) over 5-15 minutes. Angiotensin II infusion increased
aldosterone secretion only transiently during the Na replete
period, and at the start of Na depletion the rate was again basal.
Aldosterone secretion increased normally with Na depletion and fell
back to basal 3-6 hours after $NaHCO_3$ intake, despite measured sustained high blood angiotensin II levels throughout. A similar
result was obtained with homologous sheep renin infusion. The
results indicated either there was action of an unidentified agent,

or else that ionic changes had a spectacularly greater role than
hitherto attributed to them (19,29). That is, the full range of
aldosterone response to a large change of Na balance could be
caused by moderate ionic changes in the face of relatively high
blood angiotensin II levels (Fig. 3).

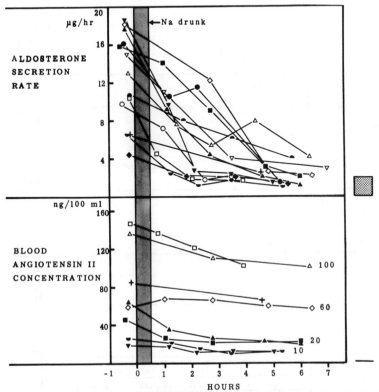

Figure 3. A series of experiments on sheep with adrenal
transplants showing the effect on aldosterone secretion
of rapid correction of body Na deficit by voluntary
drinking of 300 mEq/L NaHCO$_3$ solution. The conditions of
experiment were that the animals had been receiving a
continuous intravenous infusion of angiotensin II during
the 48 hours during which Na deficiency developed, and the
infusion was continued constant during this post drinking
phase of observation. The rates chosen for constant angiotensin II infusion in the individual experiments ranged
from 10 - 100 µg/hr which in Na replete sheep produce blood
angiotensin II levels ranging from 10 - 100 ng/100 ml -
the range seen in mild to very severe Na deficiency. Aldosterone returned to basal in normal fashion despite sustained high blood levels of angiotensin II. The normal Na
replete range of aldosterone and angiotensin II are
shown on the right.

A further series of experiments were performed in which, during the last phase - i.e., correction of Na deficiency by voluntary drinking, an intravenous infusion of KCl was begun at 6-12 mEq/hr at the time the animals began to drink. In some experiments a small increase in the rate of angiotensin II infusion was also made at this time. In some instances it was possible to prevent any overall decrease in these two factors during correction of Na deficiency. Fall of aldosterone secretion was observed under these conditions, and to an extent which was unlikely to be attributable to rise of plasma [Na] (30). Figure 4 shows such an experiment.

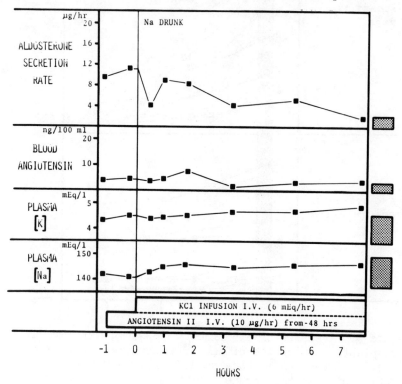

Figure 4. Ivor - adrenal transplant. The effect on aldosterone secretion of rapid correction of Na deficiency by voluntary drinking under conditions of continuous intravenous infusion of angiotensin II at constant low rate (10 µg/hr) since -48 hours, and commencement of intravenous infusion of KCl at 6 mEq/hr at the time of drinking. Aldosterone secretion fell to basal by 7 hr though blood angiotensin concentration and plasma [K] were not reduced at this time. Plasma [Na] rose. The rate of fall of aldosterone secretion to basal was retarded (cf. Fig. 3).

The rate of fall is retarded relative to control experiments where basal level is reached by 3-5 hours. However the basal secretion reached at 7 hr was not attributable to decrease of either plasma [K] or angiotensin II and was unlikely to be attributable to the small rise of plasma [Na] alone. On the other hand, the overall results under these dynamic conditions with rapidly changing extra-cellular volume and composition due to replacement of 600 - 900 mEq of Na emphasized the quantitatively large influence of changes of [K]. If the rate of KCl infusion were sufficient to produce a small [K] rise of 0.5 - 0.6 mEq/L, the decrease of aldosterone secretion following Na replacement frequently was not observed; a finding consistent with the potent effect on aldosterone secretion found with small local changes in adrenal arterial [K] (19).

In the light of this suggestive data from several experimental lines, the following experiments have been made more recently.

6.   In the studies with continuous intravenous infusion of angiotensin II no rise in renin secretion occurred in the first 24 hours of Na depletion - i.e., the angiotensin II infusion inhibited the renin release. Thus cannulae were implanted in the renal arteries of uninephrectomized sheep. Infusion at 3 µg/hr of angiotensin II did not affect systemic blood angiotensin II level in the conscious sheep - the peptide being metabolized in passage across the kidney. Over 24 hours of Na depletion, aldosterone secretion rose normally (Fig. 5). The infusion of angiotensin II inhibited the rise in systemic renin and angiotensin II. Mean plasma [K] in this series decreased 0.48 mEq/L and the small fall of plasma [Na] (mean decrease 4.2 mEq/L) was unlikely to have accounted for the extent of increase of aldosterone.

7.   Complete renal denervation has been shown to substantially abolish the increase in renin levels usually observed following Na restriction (31,32). Subsequent to denervation of the remaining kidney of uninephrectomized sheep, we have observed that the renin response to the onset of Na deficiency is impaired. Blood aldosterone concentration rose normally in response to Na deficiency. Instances were observed in the series (Fig. 6) where aldosterone response to Na deficiency could not have been attributed to increase of angiotensin II, [K], or ACTH, and the effect was greater than could be accounted for by change of plasma [Na].

8.   Concerning functional integration of central nervous mechanisms of aldosterone control, there is extremely interesting new data.

We have reported often over some years that in sheep with adrenal transplants the consummatory act of rapid satiation of

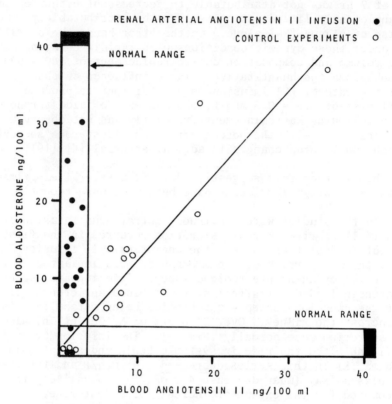

Figure 5. The effect in 8 experiments on 4 uninephrectomized
sheep of renal arterial infusion of angiotensin II at 3 µg/hr
during the onset of Na deficiency (●). Control experiments
on the relation between blood angiotensin II concentration
and blood aldosterone concentration with onset of Na deficiency
are shown (0). In experiments with renal arterial infusion
of angiotensin II (●) aldosterone increased with Na deficiency
without increase of angiotensin II concentration beyond the
normal Na replete range. In contrast to the highly significant
correlation (p<0.001) between angiotensin II and aldosterone
in the control experiments (0) there was no significant
correlation (p>0.05) between these two variables during renal
arterial angiotensin II infusion. Plasma renin levels were
normal throughout the experiment. With Na deficiency the
mean plasma [K] decreased 0.48 mEq/L (p<0.01), and the mean
plasma [Na] 4.2 mEq/L (p<0.001).

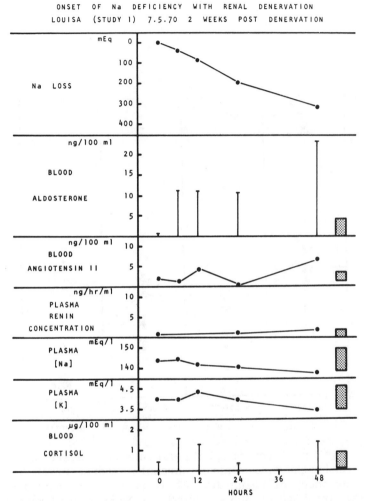

Figure 6. Louisa - renal denervation of sole kidney at -14 days. The effect of onset of Na deficiency on peripheral blood aldosterone and cortisol concentration, plasma [K] and [Na], blood angiotensin II and plasma renin concentration.

of salt appetite may cause a large evanescent decrease of aldosterone secretion over 15-30 minutes (33,34). The effect reverses
over one hour, and subsequently aldosterone falls as a result of
absorption from the gut of the Na drunk (Fig. 7).

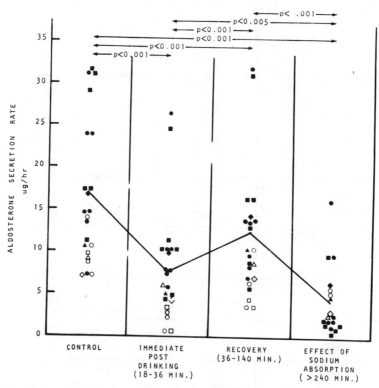

Figure 7. The effect in 22 experiments on aldosterone
secretion by the transplanted adrenal gland of 8 Na
deficient sheep of voluntary satiation of salt appetite
by rapid drinking of 300 - 900 mEq of $NaHCO_3$ solution
(300 mEq/L). The data shows a highly significant
($p < .001$ - paired t. test) decrease of mean aldosterone
secretion by 50% within 18 - 36 minutes of beginning
drinking, a highly significant partial recovery ($p < .001$)
towards control pre-drinking level by 36 - 140 minutes,
and a highly significant ($p < .001$) later fall, relative
to the 36 - 140 minute observations, due to absorption
from the gut of a substantial amount of the $NaHCO_3$
solution drunk. Mean values are shown by the solid line.

The effect is not seen in all animals, but is consistently
reproducible in the animals showing it. The rapid inhibition does
not occur if the Na is administered by tube into the rumen
(Fig. 8) and it appears that the central nervous events are
directly determinant of the phenomenon.

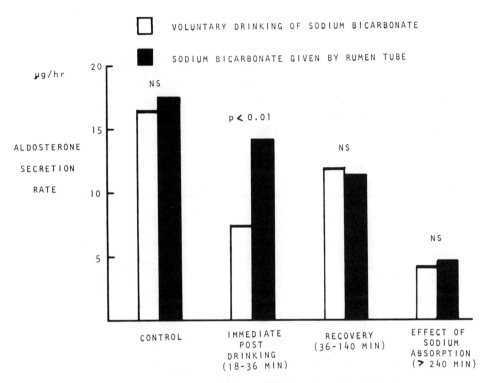

Figure 8. Comparison of the effect on mean aldosterone
secretion rate of correction of Na deficiency by voluntary drinking of $NaHCO_3$ solution (see Fig. 4) with the
effect of administering approximately the same amount
of $NaHCO_3$ into the rumen by tube. The aldosterone secretion rate at 18-36 minutes following voluntary satiation
of salt appetite was highly significantly less ($p < .01$)
than with rumen tube.

Recently with the advent of the radioimmunoassay of angiotensin II,
it has been possible formally to examine this phenomenon much
more closely. It has become unequivocally clear that a 40-50%
decrease of aldosterone secretion may occur without change of
angiotensin II, [K] or [Na]. Furthermore (Fig. 9) the effect has
been demonstrated under conditions of long continuous infusion of

angiotensin II and intravenous KCl infusion as described in
Section (5) above. The technique has been to begin intravenous
KCl infusion at the time of drinking and sometimes make a small increase in rate of angiotensin II infusion so that the fall of
aldosterone is seen under conditions where plasma [K] and blood
angiotensin II concentration are constant or even slightly
increased and [Na] unchanged. Cortisol secretion rates were
usually low and there was frequently no change associated with the
effect.

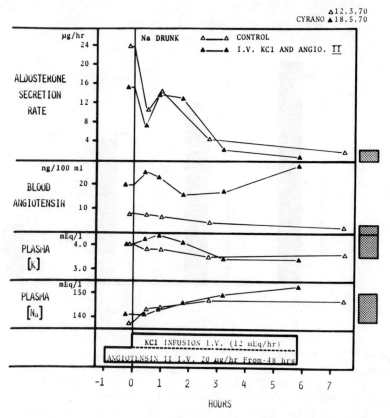

Figure 9. Cyrano - adrenal transplant - Na deficient.
The effect on aldosterone secretion rate, plasma [K],
[Na] and blood angiotensin II concentration of rapid
voluntary drinking of 900 mEq of NaHCO$_3$ solution. A
control experiment ($\triangle$ ——— $\triangle$) is compared with an
experiment ($\blacktriangle$ ——— $\blacktriangle$) where an intravenous angiotensin II infusion at 20 µg/hr, begun at -48 hr when
Na deficiency commenced, was continued at constant
rate after drinking and an intravenous KCl infusion
(12 mEq/hr) was begun also as drinking commenced.

Other experiments have been made in which the region of the adrenal transplant has been infiltrated with procaine. Also, a slow adrenal arterial infusion of hypertonic NaCl has been begun before drinking to eliminate the possibility that the effect was due to exquisite sensitivity of the adrenal to the first influx of Na into the circulation (Figure 10). In both cases the "psychic inhibition" occurred as under control conditions. In our view, this data clearly shows the existence of an unidentified humoral factor which can have a large effect on aldosterone secretion. It may involve sudden withdrawal of a stimulating factor or secretion of an inhibitor substance. Experiments aiming to identify the material are in progress. To date the only physiological substance we have determined to be capable of inhibiting aldosterone secretion upon adrenal arterial infusion in the Na deplete animal is prostaglandin E_1 though at this point we have no evidence that this substance is involved in the "psychic" inhibition (35).

   9. The studies of nephrectomy indicate that, with the exception of the direct action of [K] on the glomerulosa, angiotensin II is essential for normal aldosterone response to a number of stimuli. The question as to whether this role is largely permissive through provision of an early stage precursor for biosynthesis at the cholesterol-pregnenolone step, (26,36) or contributory causal, has been examined further in Na deficient nephrectomized sheep. The experiments were made 24-48 hours after nephrectomy, when aldosterone had fallen to basal and plasma [K] rise had been avoided by postoperative dietetic measures. Subsequent to Dexamethasone suppression of ACTH to basal levels, angiotensin II was infused at 1-2 µg/hr - a rate verified to give a blood level of 1-2 ng/100 ml (Figure 11). This is the range of the Na replete normal sheep. It was found that angiotensin II infusion at 2 µg/hr restored peripheral blood aldosterone level to the high Na deplete level observed before nephrectomy (37). This effect occurred without ionic change or alteration in blood cortisol level. Increasing the rate of angiotensin infusion to 20 µg/hr, which increased blood angiotensin level to ca. 20 ng/100 ml - the usual level for the degree of Na deficiency - did not cause any further increase in blood aldosterone level. The infusion of angiotensin II at 2 µg/hr in Na replete sheep with adrenal transplants was shown to cause only evanescent small increases of aldosterone secretion (Figure 12).

   In a recent monograph review Muller concluded also by doubting any simple view of the primacy of the renin-angiotensin system in control of aldosterone secretion and biosynthesis (38). The findings here (1-9) provide substantial stimulus for further investigation of the control of aldosterone. The experiments on rapid satiation of sodium appetite show an unidentified new factor in the regulatory system. Its role, if any, in adrenal response to slower changes of sodium balance or in other conditions changing aldosterone secretion remains to be defined. Also of importance, in general analysis, is

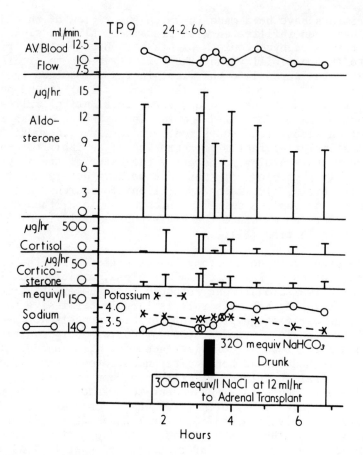

Figure 10. Adrenal transplant 9 - Na deficient. The effect
of rapid drinking of NaHCO₃ solution on the rate of aldosterone
secretion when, prior to the presentation of the solution, a
slow adrenal arterial infusion of hypertonic NaCl was commenced
to increase locally the plasma [Na] of adrenal arterial blood.
The "psychic" inhibition of aldosterone occurred as in control
experiments.

the question of the effect, if any, of changed intracellular ionic
composition of the adrenal occurring in Na deficiency on its
responsiveness to specific stimuli. We know very little about this
though the issue has been raised often during the past ten years
(30,39). Recently Davis and colleagues have published data suggesting that intracellular K content may change in Na deficiency, and
angiotensin II infusion may produce a similar effect (40). High
Na intake and plasma [Na] reduced aldosterone response to adrenal
arterial infusion of angiotensin II (23,41). The mild-moderately
Na deficient animal responds to adrenal arterial K infusion (19)

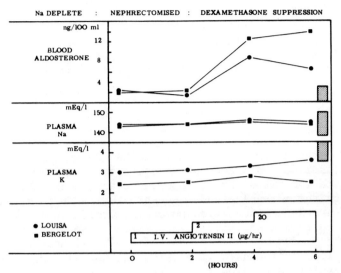

Figure 11.   Louisa and Bergolet.   Nephrectomized, Na deficient conscious sheep given Dexamethasone to suppress ACTH secretion. The effect on peripheral blood aldosterone concentration of intravenous infusion of angiotensin II at the very low rates of 1 and 2 µg/hr and at 20 µg/hr.   The plasma [Na] and [K] are shown also.   The normal Na replete range is shown on the right of the figure.

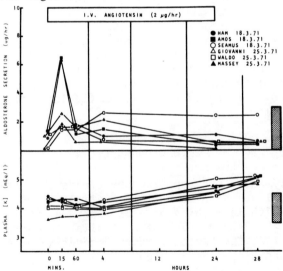

Figure 12.   The effect of intravenous infusion of angiotensin II at the low rate of 2 µg/hr for 28 hours on aldosterone secretion by the adrenal transplant of Na replete sheep. Plasma [K] is shown also.   Aldosterone hyper-secretion was not sustained.   Normal replete range is shown on the right side of the figure.

but there is little or no response to angiotensin II infusion (23).
Mild Na deficiency may increase the aldosterone response to ACTH
infusion (42,43,44).   Another facet of the control system requiring
further definition is the role, if any, of metabolites of angiotensin
II since it has been shown that the heptapeptide stimulates aldosterone secretion (45).

SUMMARY

     Study of the control of aldosterone has shown that four
factors - plasma Na and K concentration, blood angiotensin II and
ACTH concentration are of great importance and their action is
directly upon the adrenal gland.   Recent studies support earlier
evidence of another unidentified humoral factor(s) which can
influence aldosterone secretion.   Normal increase of aldosterone
secretion occurs during onset of Na deficiency without increase of
peripheral blood angiotensin II outside the normal range when renin
release is inhibited by slow renal arterial infusion of angiotensin
II.   In mild to moderate Na deficiency, infusion of angiotensin II
does not further increase aldosterone secretion whereas increase of
Na deficiency does.   In-vivo studies of aldosterone biosynthesis
during progressive Na deficiency suggest a pathway with two
components.   When aldosterone secretion is stimulated acutely by
angiotensin II the biosynthetic events do not mimic those seen in
the onset of Na deficiency.   Studies of sodium deficient animals
during and after the consummatory act of rapid satiation of salt
appetite, indicate there is a central initiated humoral mechanism
which can inhibit aldosterone secretion.   New data emphasizes the
importance of the role of small changes in plasma [K].   Questions
of the role of changed sensitivity of response of the adrenal gland
with development of Na deficiency, and the influence, if any, of the
metabolic fragments of angiotensin II, particularly the heptapeptide,
remain to be resolved.

ACKNOWLEDGEMENTS

     The work presented was supported by grants from the National
Health and Medical Research Council of Australia, the National
Institutes of Health in Washington - HE 11580-04 (GMB), the Rural
Credits Fund of the Reserve Bank of Australia, the Anti-Cancer
Council of Victoria, the National Heart Foundation of Australia
and the Australian Kidney Foundation.

REFERENCES

1. Simpson, S.A., Tait, J.R., Wettstein, A., Neher, R., von Euw, J. and Reichstein, T., Experientia, 9, 333 (1953).
2. Bartter, F.C., Mills, I., Biglieri, E.G. and Delea, C., Recent Progr. Hormone Res. 15, 311 (1959).
3. Laragh, J.H. and Stoerk, H.C., J. clin. Invest. 36, 383 (1957).
4. Wright, R.D., Med. J. Austr., 1, 88 (1961).
5. McDonald, I.R., Goding, J.R. and Wright, R.D., Austr. J. exp. Biol. med. Sci. 36, 83 (1958).
6. Denton, D.A., Goding, J.R. and Wright, R.D., Brit. med. J. ii, 447, 522 (1959).
7. Blair-West, J.R., Coghlan, J.P., Denton, D.A., Goding, J.R., Munro, J.A., Peterson, R.E. and Wintour, M., J. clin. Invest., 41, 1606 (1962).
8. Yankopoulos, N.A., Davis, J.O., Kliman, B. and Peterson, R.E., J. clin. Invest., 38, 1278 (1959).
9. Vander, A.J., Physiol. Rev., 47, 359 (1967).
10. Davis, J.O., Recent Progr. Hormone Res., 17, 293 (1961).
11. Ganong, W.F. and Mulrow, P.J., Nature, 190, 115 (1961).
12. Gross, F., Klin. Wschr., 36, 693 (1958).
13. Genest, J.E., Koiw, E., Nowaczynski, W. and Sandor, T., Abstr. First Intern. Congr. Endocrinol., 173, Denmark, 1960.
14. Laragh, J.H., Angers, M., Kelly, W.G. and Lieberman, S., J. Amer. med. Ass., 174, 234 (1960).
15. Davis, J.O., Ayers, C.R. and Carpenter, C.C.J., J. clin. Invest. 40, 1466 (1961).
16. Blair-West, J.R., Coghlan, J.P., Denton, D.A., Goding, J.R., Wintour, M. and Wright, R.D., Aust. J. exp. Biol. med. Sci., 46, 295 (1968).
17. Brown, J.J., Davies, D.L., Lever, A.F., Robertson, J.I.S., and Peart, W.S., in Baulieu and Robel Aldosterone, 417 (Blackwell Scientific Publications, Oxford 1964).
18. Gocke, D.A., Gerten, J., Sherwood, L.M. and Laragh, J.H., Circulat. Res. 24-25, Suppl. 1, 131 (1969).
19. Blair-West, J.R., Cain, M., Catt, K.J., Coghlan, J.P., Denton, D.A., Funder, J.W., Scoggins, B.A. and Wright, R.D., Proc. 3rd Int. Congr. Endocrin. Mexico, 1968, 267 (Excerpta Medica Amsterdam, 1969).
20. Binnion, P.R., Davis, J.O., Brown, T.D. and Olichney, M.J., Amer. J. Physiol., 208, 655 (1965).
21. Blair-West, J.R., Coghlan, J.P., Denton, D.A., Scoggins, B.A., Wintour, E.M. and Wright, R.D., Steroids, 15, 433 (1969).
22. Blair-West, J.R., Coghlan, J.P., Denton, D.A., Goding, J.R., Orchard, E., Scoggins, B.A., Wintour, M. and Wright, R.D., Proc. 3rd Int. Congr. Nephrol. Washington, 1966, 1, 201 (Karger, Basel/New York 1967).
23. Blair-West, J.R., Coghlan, J.P., Denton, D.A., Scoggins, B.A., Wintour, E.M., Wright, R.D., Aust. J. Exp. Biol. med. Sci. 48, 253 (1970).

24. Blair-West, J.R., Brodie, A., Coghlan, J.P., Denton, D.A.,
    Flood, C., Goding, J.R., Scoggins, B.A., Tait, J.F., Wintour,
    E.M. and Wright, R.D., J. Endocrin., 46, 453 (1970).
25. Baniukiewicz, S., Brodie, A., Flood, C., Motta, M., Okamoto,
    M., Gut, M., Tait, J.F., Tait, S.A.S., Blair-West, J.R.,
    Wintour, M. and Wright, R.D., in Functions of the Adrenal
    Cortex, 1, 153 (Appleton-Century-Crofts, New York, 1968).
26. Kaplan, N.M., J. clin. Invest., 44, 2029 (1965).
27. Blair-West, J.R., Cain, M.D., Catt, K.J., Coghlan, J.P.,
    Denton, D.A., Funder, J.W., Scoggins, B.A. and Wright, R.D.,
    Acta. Endocrin., 66, 229 (1971).
28. Blair-West, J.R., Coghlan, J.P., Denton, D.A., Funder, J.W.,
    Scoggins, B.A. and Wright, R.D., Acta. Endocrin., 66, 448
    (1971).
29. Blair-West, J.R., Cain, M., Catt, K.J., Coghlan, J.P., Denton,
    D.A., Funder, J.W., Scoggins, B.A., Wintour, E.M. and Wright,
    R.S., Proc. 4th Int. Congr. of Nephrol. Stockholm, 1969, 1,
    33 (Karger, Basel/New York 1970).
30. Blair-West, J.R., Coghlan, J.P., Denton, D.A., Goding, J.R.,
    Wintour, M. and Wright, R.D., Aust. J. exp. Biol. med. Sci.,
    44, 455 (1966).
31. Vander, A.J. and Luciano, J.R., Circulat. Res. 21, Suppl. 11,
    69 (1967).
32. Mogil, R.A., Itskovitz, J.D., Russel, J.H. and Murphy, J.J.,
    Invest. Urol. 7, 442 (1970).
33. Blair-West, J.R., Boyd, G.W., Coghlan, J.P., Denton, D.A.,
    Goding, J.R., Wintour, M. and Wright, R.D., Proc. 23rd Int.
    Congr. Physiol. Sci. Tokyo 1965, 207 (Excerpta Medica,
    Amsterdam, 1966).
34. Denton, D.A., Physiol. Rev., 45, 80 (1965).
35. Blair-West, J.R., Coghlan, J.P., Denton, D.A., Funder, J.W.,
    Scoggins, B.A. and Wright, R.D., Endocrinology, 88, 367 (1971).
36. Davis, W.W., Burwell, L.R., Kelley, G., Casper, A.G.T. and
    Bartter, F.C., Biochem. biophys. Res. Commun., 22, 218 (1966).
37. Blair-West, J.R., Cain, M.D., Catt, K.J., Coghlan, J.P.,
    Denton, D.A., Funder, J.W., Scoggins, B.A., Stockigt, J.R. and
    Wright, R.D., Proc. 3rd Int. Steroid Hormone Conf. (Hamburg
    1970).
38. Muller, J., in Regulation of Aldosterone Biosynthesis
    (Springer-Verlag, Berlin, 1971).
39. Blair-West, J.R., Coghlan, J.P., Denton, D.A., Goding, J.R.,
    Wintour, M. and Wright, R.D., Recent Progr. in Hormone Res.,
    19, 311 (1963).
40. Baumber, J.S., Davis, J.O., Johnson, A. and Witty, R.T., Amer.
    J. Physiol. 220, 1094 (1971).
41. Blair-West, J.R., Coghlan, J.P., Denton, D.A., Goding, J.R.,
    Wintour, M. and Wright, R.D., Circulat. Res. 17, 386 (1965).
42. Kinson, G.A. and Singer, B., Endocrinology, 83, 1108 (1968).

43. Williams, G.H., Dluhy, R.G. and Underwood, R.H., Clin. Sci.,
    39, 489 (1970).
44. Ganong, W.F., Biglieri, E.G. and Mulrow, P.J., Recent Progr.
    Hormone Res., 22, 381 (1966).
45. Blair-West, J.R., Coghlan, J.P., Denton, D.A., Funder, J.W.,
    Scoggins, B.A. and Wright, R.D., J. Clin. Endocrinol. 32, 575
    (1971).

EARLY MORNING VARIATION IN PLASMA RENIN ACTIVITY IN NORMAL, RECUMBENT HUMANS

M.H. Weinberger, D.R. Rosner, D.C. Kem, L. Joyner and
G. Foust

Renal-Hypertension Laboratory, Department of Medicine,
Indiana University School of Medicine, Indianapolis,
Indiana, Department of Medicine, Southwestern Medical
School, Dallas, Texas and Department of Medicine,
Tripler Army Hospital, Honolulu, Hawaii

I should like to discuss with you some interesting preliminary clinical observations. As part of a larger study involving the interaction between renin and adrenal and pituitary hormones in normal humans and hypertensive subjects, we have had the opportunity to study plasma renin levels in normal recumbent humans at 20 minute intervals in the early morning hours during normal and low dietary sodium intake. This study has yielded interesting results in terms of the concepts of diurnal rhythmicity, demonstrated by others for plasma renin activity (1).

Four normal human volunteers were studied during recumbent posture begun at 10 PM the night before. Subjects 1 and 2 were studied while ingesting a normal sodium diet; subjects 3 and 4 received a 10 mEq/d sodium intake for 3 days before the study and hydrochlorothiazide 50 mg/d on the first and second days. An indwelling venous catheter was used to obtain blood samples for plasma renin activity every 20 minutes from 2 AM to 8 AM. Blood was collected in iced vacutainer tubes with EDTA as anticoagulant and immediately centrifuged. Plasma renin activity was measured by the radio-immunoassay technique of Haber et al. (2). All samples from each subject were run as one batch.

189

Figure 1 illustrates the results obtained. Extreme variation in plasma renin activity was noted in every case. Lower values were seen in the subjects ingesting a normal sodium diet than those on salt-restricted diets. Subject 3 slept soundly throughout the study. Subjects 2 and 4 slept little because of discomfort at the catheter site. Subject 1 slept soundly until 6 AM when the catheter was re-implanted. Although a discernible peak of plasma renin activity occurred at 6 AM in this subject, it would appear from the previous sample that this peak was not related to the stress of venipuncture.

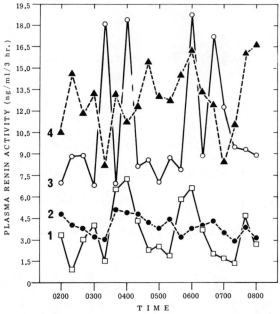

Figure 1.   Variations in plasma renin activity in four normal human volunteers recumbent from 10 PM to 8 AM. Blood samples were obtained from an indwelling catheter at 20 minute intervals from 2 AM to 8 AM.

Endogenous or pre-formed angiotensin I, represented by the samples of plasma kept at 4°C for 3 hours, when little angiotensin I generation occurs, show variations that parallel those obtained from plasma incubated at 37°C for 3 hours. Duplicate aliquots for plasma renin activity were assayed on subject 3, three months after the initial measurement with exact replication of the cyclical pattern initially observed.

Figure 2 depicts a different analysis of the data in an attempt to discern a consistent pattern of plasma renin activity among the patients studied. For each patient a mean value was determined for

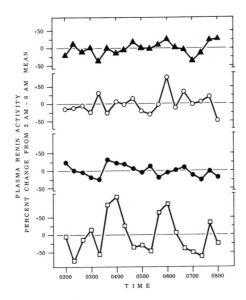

Figure 2.   Data from each patient in Figure 1 is presented as
            percent deviation from the mean of all samples ob-
            tained from a given patient (see text). No consistent
            pattern was detected.

all samples obtained and each sample was plotted as percent deviation from that mean. No consistent pattern was detected for the
patients studied.

     In 2 patients serum sodium and potassium measurements, taken
simultaneously, failed to reveal significant changes. The patients
received no food during the study and it appears unlikely that significant changes in renal tubular sodium delivery, macula densa
sodium concentration or renal perfusion pressure occurred during
the study.

     The implications of these observations are unclear. Perhaps
the observed episodic secretion of cortisol (3) and growth hormone
(4) bear analogies to bursts of renin release.

REFERENCES

1. Gordon, R.D., Wolfe, L.K., Island, D.P. and G.W. Liddle, J. Clin.
   Invest. 45:1587, 1966.
2. Haber, E., Koerner, T., Page, L.B., Kliman, B. and A. Purnode,
   J. Clin. Endocr. 29:1349, 1969.
3. Nichols, C.T. and F.H. Tyler, Ann. Rev. Med. 18:313, 1967.
4. Takahashi, Y., Kipnis, D.M. and W.H. Daughaday, J. Clin. Invest.
   47:2079, 1968.

THE RENIN-ANGIOTENSIN SYSTEM IN PATIENTS RECEIVING CHRONIC
HEMODIALYSIS

M.D. Blaufox, A. Goodman, S. Weseley, H. Schechter

and E. Weinstein

Departments of Medicine and Radiology, Albert Einstein

College of Medicine, Bronx, New York and the Renal

Laboratory, Grasslands Hospital, Valhalla, New York

The renin-angiotensin system has received comparatively little attention in chronic renal disease until this past year.
Tu (1,2) reported in 1965 that renin activity usually is low in
renal failure except in cases of acute tubular necrosis in which
marked elevations of peripheral renin activity may occur. Increased levels of renin substrate have been noted in chronic
renal disease (3) presumably reflecting decreased renin activity
and consequent reduced substrate utilization. The occurrence
of other abnormalities of the renin-angiotensin system in renal
disease also have been reported including both increased and
decreased inhibition of angiotensin generation by the plasma of
uremic patients (4,5). During the past year investigations into
this problem have been reported which are slightly at variance
but all of which agree that the severely diseased "end stage"
kidney maintains its ability to secrete renin (6,7,8,9,10,11) and
that excessive levels of renin activity may be associated occasionally with refractory hypertension in patients receiving chronic
hemodialytic treatment. The present study was performed to further evaluate renin activity, renin substrate and renin inhibitory
activity in the peripheral plasma of chronic dialysis patients
including four with "refractory hypertension."

METHODS

Seventeen patients with end-stage renal diseases are included

193

in this study. Eight subjects were maintained twice weekly at
Van Etten Hospital with chronic dialysis on the chronic twin coil
and nine were treated at Grasslands Hospital with the Kiil Dialyzer. Each patient was studied pre- and post-dialysis. Peripheral
arterial blood samples (15-20 ml) were obtained in each subject in
the morning immediately before dialysis or the day before dialysis
after the patient had remained supine for three hours and then
after 10 minutes and 1 1/2 hours in the upright position with
free activity. Post-dialysis samples were obtained in each individual after the patient had continued to remain supine for 1 1/2
hours following completion of the dialysis and then 10 minutes
and 1 1/2 hours after assuming the upright position with free
activity. Each blood sample was collected in an iced tube containing ammoniated EDTA and the plasma was immediately separated
and adjusted to pH 5.5. The samples were then frozen and assayed
later for renin activity by the method of Boucher (12) as modified
by Hickler (13). Aliquots of the supine pre- and post-dialysis
samples were used to determine substrate levels and inhibitor
activity in 10 of the "normotensive" patients and in all four
patients with refractory hypertension.

Substrate was measured using two samples each containing
one half ml of plasma incubated with 0.5 mg of a standardized
mixture of human renin (the human renin was supplied courtesy of
Dr. B. Warren) (14) for 6 hours and for 24 hours in the presence
of one ml of Dowex. This amount of renin permitted complete
substrate utilization in 6 hours. Plasma samples also were obtained from nine normal persons to establish normal substrate
values for this laboratory. In all cases the angiotensin generation at 6 hours and at 24 hours was not significantly different.
The means differed by only a few nanograms and there was no significant difference by paired t-test.

The effect of aliquots of the patient's plasma on renin activity (angiotensin generation) was determined by adding 2 ml of
pre- or post-dialysis plasma to 0.2 mg of human renin and 50 mg
of dog plasma substrate. The dog substrate was prepared in the
manner described by Boucher (15). This mixture was incubated for
4 hours in the presence of 2 ml of Dowex to determine angiotensin
generation. Six normal human plasma samples were used as controls.
This amount of renin and substrate was shown to generate angiotensin at maximum velocity during the time of incubation in the presence of normal plasma.

After incubation of each sample the angiotensin was eluted
from the Dowex in the same manner as for determining peripheral
plasma renin activity both for the inhibitor and substrate methods.
Each sample of angiotensin was assayed by two different technicians
in two different rats after coding. Results were rejected if dupli-
cates disagreed by more than 15 per cent and the samples were

reanalyzed. The normal subjects received regular diets with no medications, all were normotensive without history or evidence of renal disease.

Four of the patients included in the study had severe hypertension and all of the patients and their presumed diseases and blood pressures are listed in Table I. In five of the patients antihypertensive therapy was considered to be essential and was continued throughout the study.

The four patients who are grouped as refractory hypertensives were so designated by their personal physicians without prior knowledge of the results of the renin determinations. The remaining patients are designated "normotensive" because they were either readily controlled by hemodialysis or by modest drug therapy. Two of the hypertensive patients underwent bilateral nephrectomy during the study with excellent amelioration of their hypertension. In one of the nephrectomy patients, the disappearance of renin from the plasma was followed during surgery. No peripheral renin activity was detectable a few days after nephrectomy. The other two hypertensive patients are currently receiving frequent dialysis and intensive oral antihypertensive medication. Patients' weights were recorded but were too variable to permit meaningful interpretation. Weight gain did not correlate with degrees of hypertension.

RESULTS

Peripheral plasma renin activity in the four patients considered to have refractory hypertension was significantly higher than in the remaining chronic dialysis patients. The values obtained for the parameters studied in the hypertensive individuals are given in Table II. No standard deviation is given because of the small number of individuals. Pre-dialysis renin activity ranged from 0 to 1459 ng Angiotensin II/100 ml (ngAII%) in the thirteen "normotensive" subjects. The mean renin activity was 344 ± 118 ngAII% (SE) supine, 377 ± 114 ngAII% after 10 minutes erect and 354 ± 108 ngAII% after 1 1/2 hours in the erect position with unlimited activity. Post-dialysis the values were 442 ± 135 ngAII% (SE), 515 ± 171 ngAII% and 518 ± 173 ngAII% respectively (Figure 1). The post-dialysis renin activity was significantly higher than pre-dialysis (analyzed by the paired t test) after standing 10 minutes ($p < 0.05$) and after standing 1 1/2 hours ($p < 0.025$). Although no significant postural change occurred in peripheral renin activity pre-dialysis (paired t test), there was a significant postural effect post-dialysis at 10 minutes ($p < 0.0125$) and at 1 1/2 hours ($p < 0.025$). This postural effect was quite blunted though since normal and hypertensive subjects

TABLE I

Average B.P. (mmHg)

Patient	Age	Pre-Dialysis	Post-Dialysis	Clinical Diagnosis	Comments
1. CM	25	205/128	156/120	Chronic Glomerulonephritis	BP after nephrectomy 120/80
2. JDeS	30	175/124	150/114	Chronic Glomerulonephritis	Guanethidine
3. RP	50	200/104	202/105	Indeterminate	Bilateral Sympathectomy 1948
4. FS	49	140/80	130/60	Polycystic Kidney	- - - -
5. EM	51	152/108	150/96	Chronic Glomerulonephritis	- - - -
6. LS	50	130/80	130/80	Nephrosclerosis	- - - -
7. PS	30	120/80	110/70	Chronic Glomerulonephritis	- - - -
8. RP	31	116/110	118/82	Chronic Glomerulonephritis	Poor Dietary Control
9. RT	32	200/126	190/105	Chronic Glomerulonephritis	Poor Dietary Control
10. MA	48	210/110	170/90	Chronic Glomerulonephritis	Hydralazine
11. CF	27	190/100	170/80	Chronic Pyelonephritis	- - - -
12. PL	63	180/100	160/80	Henoch-Schoenlein Purpura	- - - -
13. HR	43	150/100	120/80	Chronic Glomerulonephritis	- - - -
14. JS	26	210/120	170/100	Chronic Glomerulonephritis	Methyldopa, Hydralazine
15. LT	28	170/100	150/90	Bilateral Cortical Necrosis	Methyldopa, Hydralazine
16. LV	49	180/90	150/80	Chronic Glomerulonephritis	Methyldopa
17. AF	13	190/130	210/130	Chronic Glomerulonephritis	Methyldopa, Hydralazine

Patients 1-9 were treated with the Kiil dialyzer, patients 10-17 with the twin coil.

TABLE II

Hypertensive Patients

Sample	Pre-Dialysis				Post-Dialysis			
	RP	CM	JDe'S	AF	RP	CM	JDe'S	AF
Supine Renin (ngAII%)	2169	3349	3759	5216	1556	9134	8602	6475
10' Erect Renin (ngAII%)	2338	4248	3527	5473	1520	8272	8519	--
1 1/2 hr Renin (ngAII%)	2406	4112	4962	5900	1908	5183	7615	--
Substrate (ngAII/ml)	694	808	900	948	748	890	983	--
Inhibitor (ngAII/2nl)	897	724	706	961	837	745	618	--

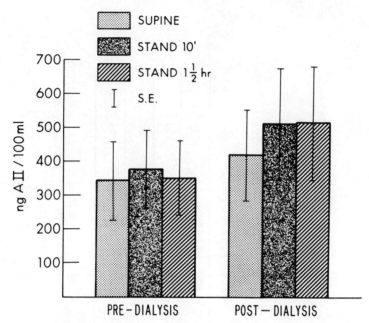

Figure 1.   The peripheral renin activity in the thirteen "normo-
             tensive" subjects is displayed as a bar graph. Note
             the slight but insignificant rise after 10 minutes
             standing pre-dialysis. After dialysis note the in-
             crease at 10 minutes but the failure to continue to
             increase at 1 1/2 hours. The values from the hyper-
             tensive subjects are in Table II.

double their peripheral renin activity after remaining 1 1/2 hours
in the upright position with unrestricted activity (Figure 2).

A significant direct linear correlation was noted between pre-
dialysis diastolic blood pressure values and pre-dialysis supine
renin activity ($r = 0.676$, $p < 0.01$) (Figure 3). There was also a
significant direct linear relationship between post-dialysis diastolic blood pressure and renin activity ($r = 0.767$, $p < 0.01$)
(Figure 4). When the pre- and post-dialysis blood pressure and
renin data were pooled and analyzed as one group, the correlation
persisted ($r = 0.593$, $p < 0.001$). No correlation could be shown
between the systolic blood pressure values and renin activity.

Renin substrate (Figure 5) in the nine normal subjects was
604 ± 146 (SD) ng AII/ml. In the 10 "normotensive" dialysis patients
studied it was 840 ± 258 ng AII/ml pre-dialysis and 770 ± 246 ng AII/ml
post-dialysis. The slight difference in the post-dialysis value
is not significant. The substrate levels in the dialysis patients,
however, were significantly higher than the normal ($p < 0.025$).
The hypertensive subjects had substrate levels which were comparable

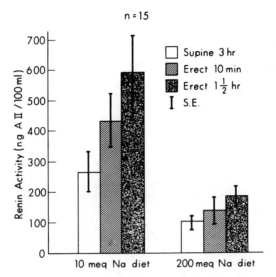

Figure 2.   Renin activity on high and low sodium intake in re-
            lation to posture is shown for fifteen patients with
            essential hypertension. Note that the supine levels
            at both intakes are lower than in the dialysis pa-
            tients (Figure 1) and the postural response is great-
            er, especially at one and a half hours.

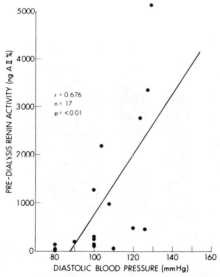

Figure 3.   Relationship between pre-dialysis renin activity and
            diastolic blood pressure at the time of the sample.
            There is a direct linear relationship between the
            pressure and the renin activity. The regression line
            is shown.

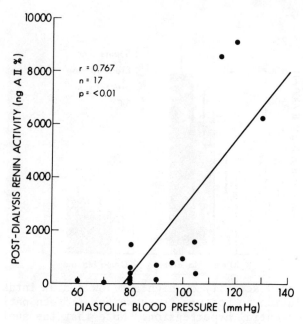

Figure 4.   Diastolic blood pressure and renin activity post-
            dialysis. Note increasing renin activity at high
            levels of blood pressure.

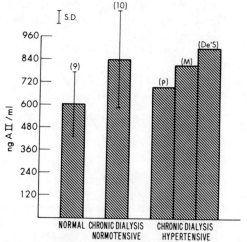

Figure 5.   Renin substrate levels expressed as ngAII/ml in normal
            subjects and in "normotensive" and hypertensive dialy-
            sis patients. The mean of the level of substrate in
            the dialysis patients is significantly higher than
            normal. The levels in the hypertensive subjects over-
            lap with the normal subjects and "normotensive" pa-
            tients. The substrate level in one of the hypertensive
            patients which is not shown was 948 ngAII/ml.

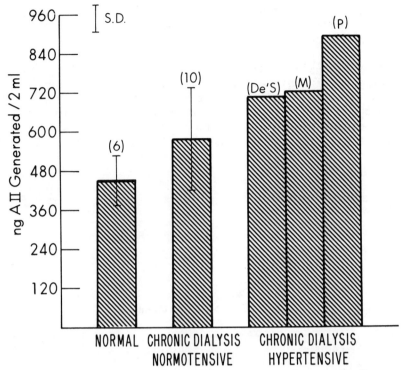

Figure 6.   Renin activity in the presence of normal plasma and
            plasma from patients receiving chronic dialysis.
            Increased angiotensin generation occurred in the
            presence of the abnormal plasma.   Inhibitor was mea-
            sured in 10 of the 13 "normotensive" patients.   The
            value for the fourth hypertensive patient who is not
            shown was 961 ngAII/2ml.

to those found in the other dialysis patients (Table II) and which
definitely were not reduced.

     Angiotensin generation in the presence of normal plasma was
highly reproducible and averaged 453 ± 71 ng AII/2ml (SD) (Figure 6).
The amount of angiotensin generated was much more variable in the
presence of the plasma of the dialysis patients and averaged
580 ± 142 ngAII/2ml pre-dialysis and 573 ± 148 ngAII/2ml post-dialysis.
There was significantly greater angiotensin generation in the
presence of the patient's plasma ($p < 0.05$).   Increased angiotensin
generation suggests decreased inhibitory activity.   The range was
417 to 840 ngAII/2ml and there was no evidence in any renal failure
patient of increased renin inhibitor activity such as has been reported in chronic glomerulonephritis (4).   The values for inhibitor in the hypertensive dialysis patients were comparable to the

values obtained in other dialysis patients. Both groups revealed increased angiotensin generation signifying decreased inhibitor or possibly a renin accelerator.

In one hypertensive patient there was an opportunity to follow the disappearance of renin activity from the plasma at the time of surgury. The time of ligation of the kidneys' arterial supply was taken as zero and blood samples were obtained at 0, 5, 10, 20, 40, 50 and 60 minutes. The data could be fitted best as a single exponential with a half time of 48 minutes. The final sample at one hour had 37% of the initial renin activity (Figure 7).

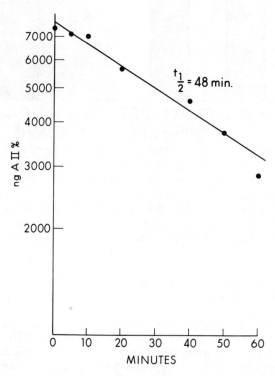

Figure 7.   The plasma disappearance of renin activity in a chronic dialysis patient with refractory hypertension (semi-logarithmic plot). Note the prolonged half time and that this is a single exponential during the first hour. Later sampling was not practical because of the patient's severe anemia. However, the next day there was no detectable renin activity in the plasma.

DISCUSSION

The ability of the severely diseased kidney to secrete renin
confirms the persistent function of this organ as an endocrine
apparatus even after excretory function is completely lost. Other
reports (1,2,8,21) have suggested that renin secretion is abnormal
in chronic renal disease and the present study reveals a blunted
but appropriate response to both postural and volume changes. The
low renin activity frequently found in chronic dialysis patients
is not surprising in view of the inability of these patients to
excrete a salt and water load.

The renin activity of patient's plasma pre-dialysis may be
compared with normal or hypertensive patients receiving a high
sodium intake (Figure 2), since these patients are probably frequently sodium loaded. In this laboratory renin activity in normal subjects in the supine, ten minute standing and 1 1/2 hour
erect positions is 117+56 ngAII% (SD), 181+84 ngAII% and 222+100
ngAII% respectively. Values for salt loaded hypertensive subjects
are slightly lower. The mean pre-dialysis supine renin activity
of 344 ngAII% with a rise to 377 ngAII% at 10 minutes and 354
ngAII% at one and one-half hours in the patients presently studied
is actually at a level higher than the normal or hypertensive salt
loaded subject. So that although there clearly is a blunted
postural response, the absolute level of renin activity pre-dialysis appears to be inappropriately high (8). Although this is true
of the mean values there is a great range of values encountered and
some of the dialysis patients do have suppressed renin activity.

Individual differences in voluntary fluid restriction may
account in part for the wide range in pre-dialysis values encountered in this study. This supposition is currently unsettled since
the recent studies of Gutkin et al (9) and of Wilkinson et al (18)
failed to demonstrate a relationship between renin activity and
plasma volume or exchangeable sodium. Support of the concept of
volume overload as a significant cause of low renin activity in
many patients with chronic renal disease is inferred from the lack
of postural response in most of these patients (8). In the present study no significant postural response was present before
dialysis in the "normotensive" patients but after dialysis there
was a definite partial restoration of a postural renin response.
This response is blunted and unsustained. At 10 minutes it is
easily detected but later samples fail to show the continued rise
in renin activity previously noted in normal subjects and in patients with essential hypertension in this laboratory (16). If
volume is suppressing renin,pre-dialysis, it only accounts partially for the values observed.

The hypertensive dialysis patients appear to react somewhat
differently, almost as if the organ were autonomously secreting

renin. All four patients show some postural response pre-dialysis
but the response is not sustained and in two of them post-dialysis
there is a postural fall in activity. This lack of postural
rise may be accounted for only partly by the relative inaccuracy
of the assay at very high levels of activity. There appears to
be a failure of the organ to maintain continuous secretion at such
high levels. This response along with the very high levels observed may help to separate out the subgroup of severely hypertensive dialysis patients which were first described by Onesti (17).

Another interesting finding is the correlation between pre-
dialysis diastolic blood pressure and renin activity and between
post-dialysis diastolic blood pressure and renin activity.
Wilkinson et al (18) failed to show a correlation between exchangeable sodium and blood pressure but did report a highly significant
correlation between diastolic blood pressure and plasma renin
activity. They also report a significant correlation between
systolic pressure and renin which this study fails to confirm.
Their measurements were taken on the day before and the day after
dialysis. These data suggest that although renin may play a role
in the regulation of diastolic blood pressure in all dialysis
patients, other factors are usually involved. One of these factors may be volume expansion. If this is true then the observation here may be explained by the rearragement of the interrela-
tionships of factors controlling the blood pressure pre- and post-
dialysis. The severely hypertensive dialysis patients may be
separated out as a group in which renin secretion is relatively
autonomous and clearly out of proportion to plasma volume and vascular tone. However, it is important to emphasize that the present data suggest these findings differ mainly in the magnitude of
the response when comparing hypertensive to "normotensive" dialysis patients.

Previous reports and the present study seem to confirm that
in at least some patients with end-stage renal disease the renin-
angiotensin system may be implicated. Yamaguchi et al (10),
Onesti (17), Brown (6), Safar et al (11) and the present study as
well as others have all noted good blood pressure control after
bilateral total nephrectomy in patients with high renin activity.
The finding of greatly increased peripheral renin activity in a
patient with refractory hypertension receiving dialytic treatment
may be an indication for consideration of bilateral nephrectomy.
The final decision would depend upon a knowledge that the patient
is receiving adequate dietary and dialytic therapy and that the
risk of his hypertension outweighs the risk of nephrectomy. The
renal source of the renin activity seems quite clear since renin
activity in the patients reported has fallen to near to zero
shortly after nephrectomy. Nephrectomy may also help to make
control of hypertension easier in patients who refuse to faith-

fully follow more conservative treatment.

The disappearance of renin activity from the plasma after
nephrectomy is also of interest. Safar et al (11) followed plasma renin for up to 5 hours in 5 patients after ligation of the
second renal pedicle. The half time of disappearance in 4 of their
cases appears to be about one hour. The case reported here would
be in reasonable agreement, and would represent a somewhat short-
er half time of disappearance of plasma renin activity than has
been suggested by Assaykeen (22) and others. No estimates of
disappearance of renin from the plasma of normal man are available for comparison, so that at present it cannot be determined
if the disappearance of renin from the plasma in these patients
is normal, shortened or prolonged.

Renin substrate is elevated in the dialysis patients included
in this study and this is in agreement with previous observations
(3). Recently however Kotchen et al (7) have reported normal substrate concentrations in patients undergoing chronic dialysis.
The substrate concentration in their patients was 963 ng/ml+
163 SD, which is actually higher than that noted in this study.
The difference in their conclusion is caused by their finding of
a higher value for normal substrate concentrations than noted in
this laboratory. Values for mean normal substrate concentrations
have been summarized by Page and McCubbin (19) for several laboratories and range from 425 ngAII/ml to 900 ngAII/ml. The average
is 705 ngAII/ml according to these authors. An increase in substrate would be expected to be related to lack of substrate utilization, increased hepatic production, or decreased metabolism.
Since uremic patients are frequently in negative protein balance,
decreased metabolism of substrate seems unlikely. Decreased utilization occasionally may be an explanation of the substrate levels
observed, but the four hypertensive patients all had levels of
substrate in the upper range of normal in spite of continued
high levels of renin activity. Also it has already been pointed
out that supine renin activity in these patients in general is
relatively high. The possibility remains that the increased substrate levels noted in these patients is related to increased hepatic synthesis. However, the lack of agreement between this
study and Kotchen's (7) may simply reflect a great variability in
normal substrate concentration. Both Kotchen's and the present
results are very much at variance with the study of Safar (11)
which reports normal substrate concentrations of 470 ng/ml.

A surprising finding is the decreased renin inhibitory activity in all of these patients. This is in contrast to the earlier
report of Maebashi (4) but in agreement with the findings of
Kotchen (7) and of Ueda (5). It is possible that this may represent decreased secretion of a renin inhibitor by the kidney as

suggested by Kotchen or that the renin inhibitors are dialyzable.
There was no difference in renin activity in the patients receiving Kiil as opposed to twin coil dialysis and no differences were
noted pre- and post-dialysis. Hoebler (19) has reported an altered substrate appearing after nephrectomy in animals. Ueda suggests
that this altered substrate with abnormal kinetics provides a possible explanation for increased renin generation in uremic plasma,
but the present study utilized the same exogenous substrate for
both uremic and normal plasma. The explanation of this phenomenon
cannot be expected until technics are available which will permit
the measurement of inhibitor in normal and uremic subjects quantitatively on a semi-routine basis.

The abnormalities of the renin-angiotensin system in end stage
renal disease as suggested in this study are multiple. Measurable
peripheral renin activity is present in most patients and responses
to volume and posture change although markedly blunted also are
present. Part of the renin activity in peripheral plasma can be
accounted for by increased substrate concentrations and decreased
renin inhibitory activity. It is noteworthy that these findings
are relatively consistent in all hemodialysis patients and that
hypertensive dialysis patients are distinguished from "normotensive" dialysis patients only by a disporportionately increased
renin activity and the other abnormalities of the system are
shared. In at least some dialysis patients renin secretion may
achieve a state vaguely akin to "tertiary hyperparathyroidism"
with the kidney secreting renin at levels which are clearly inappropriately high for the physiologic circumstances and are sustained. The possibility of prolonged half time of renin in the
plasma may make this possible even at relatively low secretion
rates when compared to normal subjects. Proper treatment for the
hypertension in some of these individuals may be total bilateral
nephrectomy. The high complication rate of nephrectomy reported
by Wilkinson (18) should be considered carefully in making this
decision. Since the vast majority of patients with chronic renal
disease who are hypertensive have relatively normal renin activity
it seems possible that the kidney may secrete another as yet unidentified pressor substance, and that the cause of the hypertension is multifactorial.

Whatever the role of the renin may be in the hypertension of
chronic renal disease, a primary role is probably uncommon.
Among the 121 patients included in this study and several others
(2,6,7,11,21) only 18 were considered to have markedly elevated
renin activity. Each of these 18 patients was categorized as a
severe or refractory hypertensive.

The exact role of the renin-angiotensin system in the hypertension encountered in end-stage renal disease cannot be evalu-

ated fully until the cause of hypertension in earlier stages of chronic renal disease is identified. Consideration must be given to the appropriateness of renin levels. That is, in a given individual the renin activity may be in the normal range but may be inappropriately high for that blood pressure or plasma volume. Continued detailed studies of the patient with obvious renin abnormalities are needed to ultimately clarify the role of renin in renal hypertension.

ACKNOWLEDGEMENTS

This work was supported in part by NIH Grants FR50 and HE11984.

The authors wish to thank Mrs. Hyo-Bok Lee, Mr. Yigal Greener, and Miss Theresa Liang for their technical assistance in the performance of this study.

REFERENCES

1. Tu, W. H. Plasma renin of advanced nephritis treated by long term hemodialysis. Clin Res 13:116, 1965.
2. Tu, W. H. Plasma renin activity in acute tubular necrosis and other renal diseases associated with hypertension. Circ 31:686-695, 1965.
3. Helmer, O.M. and Judson, W.E. The quantitative determination of renin in the plasma of patients with arterial hypertension. Circ 27:1050-1060, 1963.
4. Maebashi, M., Miura, Y., and Yoshinaga, K. Renin inhibitor in plasma of uremic patients. Lancet 1408-1409, 1968.
5. Ueda, H, Takeda, T., Kouji, N., Massao, I., and Ebihara, A. Effect of uremic human plasma on renin activity. Jap Heart J 6:416-427, 1965.
6. Brown, J.J., Curtis, J.R., Lever, A.F., Robertson, J.J.S., DeWardener, H.E. and Wing, A.J. Plasma renin concentration and the control of blood pressure in patients on maintenance hemodialysis. Nephron 6:329-349, 1969.
7. Kotchen, T.A., Knight, E.L., Kashgarian, M., and Mulrow, P.J. A study of the renin angiotensin system in patients with severe chronic renal insufficiency. Nephron 7:317-330, 1970.
8. Warren, D. and Ferris, T. Renin secretion in renal hypertension. Lancet Jan. 24:159-163, 1970.
9. Gutkin, M., Levinson, G., King, A., and Lasker, N. Plasma renin activity in end stage kidney disease. Circ 40:563-574, 1969.
10. Yamaguchi, H., Fujii, J., Seki, P., Kurihara, H., Ikeda, M., and Mimura, N. Increased plasma renin activity in chronic renal failure associated with severe hypertension: relation-

ship between plasma renin level and peritoneal dialysis.
Jap Circ J 33:63-67, 1969.

11. Safar, M., Fendler, J.P., Weil, B., Beauve, Mery, P., Brisset,
     J.M., Idatte, J.M., Meyer, P. and Milliez, P. Hypertension
     in patients on maintenance haemodialysis. Rev Europe Etudes
     Clin et Biol 15:740-747, 1970.

12. Boucher, R., Veyrat, R., deChamplain, J., and Genest, J. New
     procedures for measurement of human plasma angiotensin and
     renin activity levels. Canada M.A.J. 90:194-201, 1964.

13. Blaufox, M.D., Birbari, A., Hickler, R., and Merrill, J.P.
     Peripheral plasma renin activity in renal homotransplant
     recipients. New Engl J Med 275:1164-1168, 1966.

14. Warren, B., Johnson, A., and Hoobler, S. Characterization of
     the renin angiotensin system. J Exp Med 123:1109-1128, 1966.

15. Boucher, R., Menard, J., and Genest, J. A micromethod for
     measurement of renin in the plasma and kidney of rats. Can
     J Physiol Pharmac 45:881-890, 1967.

16. Blaufox, M.D., and Fotino, S. Renin activity in essential hyp-
     ertension. Clin Res 42:424, 1969.

17. Onesti, G., Swartz, C., Ramirez, O., and Brest, A. Bilateral
     nephrectomy for control of hypertension in uremia. Trans
     Amer Soc Artif Intern Organs 14:361, 1968.

18. Wilkinson, R., Scott, D., Uldall, P., Kerr, D., and Swinney,J.
     Plasma renin and exchangeable sodium in the hypertension of
     chronic renal failure. Quarterly J Med 39:377-394, 1970.

19. Hoobler, S., Schroeder, J., Blaquier, P., and Demerjian, Y.
     Further studies on mechanism whereby nephrectomy augments
     pressor response to renin. Can Med Assoc J 90:227, 1964.

20. Page, I., and McCubbin, J. Renal Hypertension. p. 31-33
     Yearbook Medical Publishers, Inc., Chicago, Ill., 1968.

21. Stokes, G.S., Mani, M., and Stewart, J. Relevance of salt,
     water and renin to hypertension in chronic renal failure.
     Brit Med J 3:126-129, 1970.

22. Assaykeen, T.A., Otsuka, K., and Ganong, W.F. Rate of disap-
     pearance of exogenous dog renin from the plasma of nephrecto-
     mized dogs. Proc Soc Exp Biol and Med 127:306-310, 1968.

A PARADOXICAL RESPONSE TO CHANGES IN SODIUM INTAKE IN PATIENTS WITH ACCELERATED HYPERTENSION

P.J. Mulrow, T.A. Kotchen and L.B. Morrow

Department of Internal Medicine, Yale Univeristy School

of Medicine, New Haven, Connecticut

Many investigators have reported a decrease in plasma renin activity or concentration with sodium loading and a rise following sodium deprivation (1). The present report describes a paradoxical response of plasma renin activity to changes in dietary sodium intake in 4 patients with severe hypertension.

METHODS

The patients were studied under metabolic balance conditions. They received a measured high sodium diet (250 mEq Na, 75 mEq K) for 4 to 5 days. Two of the patients were subsequently placed on a 10 mEq Na, 75 mEq K diet for 4 to 5 days. Frequent serum and urine electrolytes, BUN and creatinine clearances were measured on both diets. Plasma renin activity (PRA) both in the supine position and after four hours in the upright position, was measured on the final day of each diet. A modified Boucher technique described previously (2) was used for two patients and the Skinner method for the other two patients (3). Aldosterone excretion or secretion was measured by the double isotope method of Kliman and Peterson (4).

Of the four patients, three had renovascular hypertension (patients A, B, C). Patients A and B were subsequently cured of their hypertension by unilateral nephrectomy and patient C has been treated medically. Patient D was in the malignant phase of essential hypertension. Three of the four patients had accelerated hypertension, characterized by high pressures, renal impairment and in two patients (A and D) grade 4 retinopathy. Patient B at the time of study could not be classified as having accelerated hypertension but within 1 month was admitted with malignant hypertension

209

and grade 4 eyegrounds.

RESULTS

Figure 1 shows the effect of a high and low sodium diet on the upright plasma renin level in normal and hypertensive subjects. In both the normal subjects and the patients with benign hypertension, there was an increase in PRA on the low sodium diet. A number of the hypertensive patients had a suppressed plasma renin response to the low sodium diet but none of the normal or hypertensive subjects had a lower PRA on the low sodium diet.

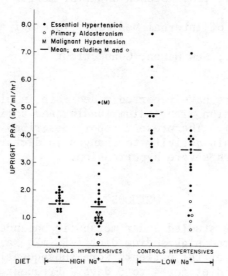

Figure 1. Upright plasma renin levels in normal and hypertensive subjects during high and low dietary sodium intake.

Figure 2 shows the typical increase in aldosterone excretion that occurs during sodium depletion. The hypertensive patients have a suppressed response in aldosterone excretion.

In contrast, in Figure 3, the four patients with severe hypertension had a paradoxical response: a lower supine PRA on the low sodium diet than on the high sodium diet. The solid lines indicate PRA measured by a modified Boucher technique in 2 patients and the dotted lines indicate the PRA measured by the Skinner technique in two patients. The dotted line connecting the 5.2 and 12.6 ng/ml/hr values shows the increase in PRA between the second and third days of the high sodium diet.

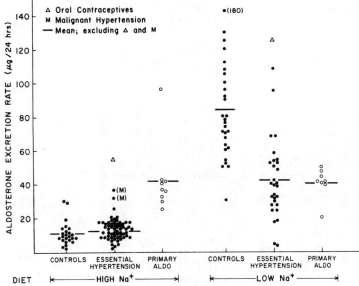

Figure 2.   Aldosterone excretion rates in normal and hypertensive subjects during high and low dietary sodium intake.

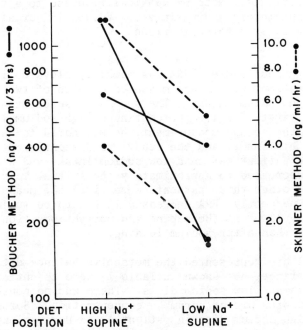

Figure 3.   Paradoxical renin response to changes in sodium intake in four patients with severe hypertension. (See text)

In Figure 4 are shown the individual PRA values obtained in the supine and erect position and the values in normal subjects for comparison.

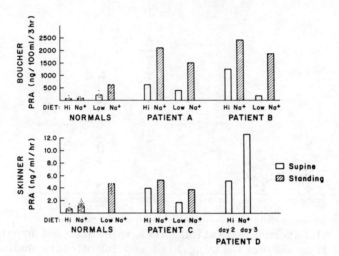

Figure 4.   Plasma renin levels in four severely hypertensive
            patients. Note paradoxical response to alterations
            in dietary sodium intake. Values in normal subjects
            are given for comparison.

On the high sodium diet, PRA was markedly elevated in all patients. In patient D, PRA was measured on each of two successive days of the high sodium intake. The second measurement was greater than twice the first, despite the continued high sodium intake. On the morning of the second measurement, he was noted to have fresh hemorrhages in his fundi, and the study was discontinued. Two weeks later while the patient was on a low sodium intake and a diuretic drug, PRA had decreased to approximately the initial value (6.1 ng/ml/hr). The other three patients were given the measured low sodium diet. Unexpectly, PRA decreased in the three subjects, and was considerably lower in the supine and upright position after sodium deprivation than after sodium loading.

In Table 1 are represented the metabolic balance data. BUN and creatinine clearance, not shown in Table 1, were essentially the same on the high and low sodium diets. There was no consistent change in blood pressure or serum Na concentration. Serum K was lower on the high sodium diet in patient A and D. Patient B was in persistent negative K balance on the high sodium diet. The only consistent finding was an increased K excretion on the high Na diet. Unlike the renin response, aldosterone excretion increased following sodium deprivation in two patients.

TABLE 1
METABOLIC BALANCE STUDIES

	Diet	PRA Supine	PRA Standing	Aldosterone (ug/24 hr)	Serum Na (mEq/L)	Serum K (mEq/L)	Urine Na (mEq/24 hr)	Urine K (mEq/24 hr)	Blood Pressure Supine (mm Hg)	Blood Pressure Standing (mm Hg)
Patient A	High Na (day 4)	635 (B)	2085	37	134	2.3	213	53	200/120	150/100
	Low Na (day 5)	400	1520	70	134	3.3	10	49	180/116	150/110
Patient B	High Na	1260 (B)	2420	27	134	–	209	81	200/110	–
	Low Na	162	1882	–	138	3.9	14	54	190/130	–
Patient C	High Na (day 4)	4.0 (S)	5.3	8	141	4.7	230	66	194/156	200/140
	Low Na (day 4)	1.7	3.8	24	139	4.9	46	52	200/150	226/162
Patient D	High Na (day 2)	5.2 (S)	–	34	137	3.4	140	61	230/150	–
	High Na (day 3)	12.6	–	–	139	3.2	419	83	200/150	–

(B) Boucher Method ng/100 ml/3 hr   (S) Skinner Method ng/ml/hr

DISCUSSION

Several unusual features of the renin-aldosterone system are demonstrated in these patients with severe hypertension. In contrast to normal subjects, and patients with benign hypertension, in whom sodium loading suppresses and sodium deprivation stimulates renin and aldosterone secretion, we have observed that sodium loading paradoxically stimulates renin secretion. Furthermore, although PRA decreased following sodium deprivation, aldosterone excretion increased appreciably. Of over 40 hypertensive patients evaluated according to a similar protocol, these were the only four patients with the paradoxical response. Three of these patients had accelerated hypertension. The other patient (patient B in Table 1) was a woman with renovascular hypertension and blood pressure in the range of 200/130 mm Hg. She was in negative potassium balance on the high sodium diet. One month later, she presented in malignant hypertension with grade 4 hypertensive retinopathy. Unilateral nephrectomy cured the hypertension. Only one other patient with accelerated hypertension was studied on this protocol and he had the normal response to changes in sodium intake. This abnormal response is not peculiar to patients with renovascular hypertension since most patients with the benign form of this hypertension have normal PRA on a high sodium diet (5).

The mechanism of this paradoxical renin response is not at all clear. One possibility is that the renin response may be an early sign of renal ischemia associated with the necrotizing arteritis of accelerated hypertension which was aggravated by sodium loading. The appearance of fresh hemorrhages in the fundi of patient D supports this possibility, but there was no decrease in creatinine clearance or change in blood pressure. In this patient a pronounced spontaneous natriuresis occurred which lasted one day. Perhaps this natriuresis was the cause of the elevated PRA. However, two weeks later while he was on a low sodium intake and a diuretic drug, PRA had returned to the lower value on day 3.

Potassium deficiency has been reported to stimulate PRA and suppress aldosterone production while K loading decreases PRA and stimulates aldosteronism (6,7,8,9). Conceivably, our finding of an elevated PRA associated with a high sodium intake and the dissociation between the renin and aldosterone responses might be related to changes in K balance. The enhanced potassium excretion due to the secondary aldosteronism associated with malignant hypertension is further augmented by the high sodium intake. On the high sodium diet, patient A was clearly hypokalemic. At the completion of the low sodium diet, serum K had increased from 2.8 mEq/L to 3.3 mEq/L and, although aldosterone excretion rose to 70 μg/24 hr, PRA was considerably lower than it had been on the high sodium diet. Similarly, patient D demonstrated a rising PRA on the high sodium intake at a time when serum K was falling and there was evidence of urinary K wasting. There was also evidence of negative K balance in patient B on a high sodium diet.

Patient C, however, had no evidence of K depletion, but K excretion on the high sodium diet was greater than on the low sodium diet. If the unusual renin responses are related to changes in K balance the K alterations may be more subtle than changes in serum K concentration. Indeed, in both the human and the rat, intracellular K rather than serum K seems to be the important parameter affecting aldosterone secretion (10,11).

Another interpretation of the K data is that a relative K loading during sodium deprivation suppresses plasma renin activity.

SUMMARY

A paradoxical response in PRA to sodium loading and deprivation occurred in 4 patients with severe hypertension. The possible relationship of this response to the potassium balance is discussed.

REFERENCES

1. Mulrow, P.J., 1969, Aldosterone in hypertension and edema. In: Duncan's Diseases of Metabolism, ed. P.K. Bondy, W.B. Saunders Co. 20: 1083-1102.
2. Gorden, P., Ferris, T., and Mulrow, P., 1967, Rabbit uterus as a possible site of renin synthesis, Am. J. Physiol. 212:703-706.
3. Skinner, S.L., 1967, Improved assay methods for renin concentration and activity in human plasma, Circulation 20:391-402.
4. Kliman, B. and Peterson, R.E., 1960, Double isotope derivative assay of aldosterone in biological extracts, J. Biol. Chem. 235: 1639-1648.
5. Kotchen, T.A., Lytton, B., Morrow, L.B., Mulrow, P.J., Shutkin, P.M., and Stansel, H.C., 1970, Angiotensin and aldosterone in renovascular hypertension, Arch. Intern. Med. 125:265-272.
6. Sealey, J.E., Clark, I., Bull, M.B., and Laragh, J.H., 1970, Potassium balance and the control of renin secretion, J. Clin. Invest. 49:2119-2127.
7. Brunner, H.R., Baer, L., Sealey, J.E., Ledingham, J.G., and Laragh, J.H., 1970, The influence of potassium administration and potassium deprivation on plasma renin in normal and hypertensive subjects, J. Clin. Invest. 49:2128-2138.
8. Veyrat, R., Brunner, H.R., Manning, E.L., and Muller, A.F., 1967, Inhibition de l'activite' lat renine plasmatique par le potassium, J. Urol. Nephrol. 73:271.
9. Vander, A.J., 1970, Direct effects of potassium on renin secretion and renal function, Am. J. Physiol. 219:455-459.

10. Boyd, J.E., Palmore, W.P., and Mulrow, P.J., 1971, Potassium,
     is it the adrenal glomerulotrophin ?, J. Clin. Invest. 50:35
     (Abstract)

11. Cannon, P.J., Ames, R.P., and Laragh, J.H., 1966, Relation
     between potassium balance and aldosterone secretion in normal
     subjects and in patients with hypertensive or renal tubular
     disease, J. Clin. Invest. 45:865-879.

LOW PLASMA RENIN IN HYPERTENSIVE PATIENTS: CORRELATIONS WITH

ALDOSTERONE, SODIUM AND POTASSIUM EXCRETION

J.A. Luetscher and R. Beckerhoff

Department of Medicine, Stanford University School of

Medicine, Stanford, California

Physicians have learned much from physiological studies of the control of renin and aldosterone secretion, but our understanding of the variations in circulating hormones in patients with hypertension is still far from complete. This paper will describe some aspects of low plasma renin activity (PRA) in hypertensive patients.

Low PRA in primary aldosteronism was predicted as a result of negative feedback and was demonstrated by several research teams (1 to 4). Patients with primary aldosteronism do not increase PRA to a normal extent after standing and in moderate sodium depletion (5). Brown (4) and Helmer (6) found an unexpectedly high incidence of suppressed renin activity in essential hypertension. It is now generally accepted that one-fourth of all patients with essential hypertension have suppressed plasma renin activity (7). The incidence of low PRA greatly exceeds that of primary aldosteronism, and indeed, most low-renin hypertensives do not have demonstrable hyperaldosteronism. In these cases, PRA responds sub-normally to salt deprivation and to the upright posture, or to a drug-induced fall in blood pressure (7,8,9). If sufficiently prolonged and severe sodium depletion is induced, and particularly if potassium depletion follows diuretic administration, a considerable rise in plasma renin activity can be stimulated (8). In all of these respects, the low-renin hypertensive resembles the patient with primary aldosteronism, but the degree of renin suppression is greater in hyperaldosteronism and maximal in cases with adenoma (Table 1).

In the earlier reports, suppression of plasma renin activity was commonly demonstrated after several days on a low sodium diet,

218

J.A.LUETSCHER AND R. BECKERHOFF

TABLE I

Plasma Renin Concentration in
Low-Renin Hypertensives with Hyperaldosteronism

Sodium Intake	High		Low	
Posture	Lying	Standing	Lying	Standing
No tumor	3.83	4.82	4.90	5.43
Tumor	1.85	2.24	3.55	3.78

Analysis of Variance (Rows) F = 10.5, p < .01

when the normal rise in PRA was significantly greater than that of the low-renin cases. The low-renin group were therefore designated "non-responders" (7,8,10). With the development of more sensitive methods, the plasma renin concentration in these patients can be shown to be subnormal on either a high or a low-sodium diet (Table 1). We will refer to these cases simply as low-renin hypertensives. Substrate concentration is generally normal in these individuals and there is no evidence of alteration in co-factors (8,10).

Woods and Liddle (11) and Jose, Crout and Kaplan (7) have shown a significant expansion of extracellular fluid volume and exchangeable sodium in the patient with low PRA, as compared with control hypertensive patients. Weinberger et al. (8) showed that the low renin hypertensives lost more sodium and had a greater fall in blood pressure during sodium depletion by diet and diuretics than other hypertensives. When the initially higher extracellular fluid volume is corrected for the greater sodium loss during dietary deprivation, it appears that the sodium status of the low renin hypertensive reaches a level approximately equivalent to that of the other hypertensive patients who take a low sodium diet. In order to explain the continuing suppression of renin on the low sodium diet, it is necessary to assume that some additional factor above and beyond the extracellular fluid volume and exchangeable sodium must be acting to prevent the expected rise in PRA. It would seem, therefore, that we are dealing with at least two anomalies in the low-renin patient. First, he has an unusually high extracellular fluid volume and exchangeable sodium on a normal or high sodium intake, and second, his PRA fails to respond normally to sodium depletion.

In order to investigate the nature of these anomalous responses, we have stressed the control mechanism, first, by very heavy sodium loading (diet plus added sodium 300 mEq per day) and have followed this with 5 to 7 days on a low-sodium diet (10 mEq per day). We have compared normotensive controls, patients with hypertension and various levels of PRA, categorized as high, normal and low. Measurements of PRA have been summarized in a recent paper (12) and supplemented by measurements of plasma renin concentration (PRC).

It has been repeatedly and correctly stated that most hypertensive patients have normal aldosterone secretion rate on a normal sodium intake. When sodium intake is very high, however, many hypertensive patients continue to secrete and excrete approximately the same quantity of aldosterone as on a normal sodium intake, while in normal individuals the high sodium intake causes a considerable suppression of aldosterone production. The relationship between plasma renin activity and aldosterone is very strong in normal men, and a similar relationship exists between PRA and aldosterone in many hypertensive patients. Only in the low-renin group does a marked dissociation between PRA and aldosterone production occur (12). The abnormality in the low-renin cases consists of a higher than normal basal aldosterone production in relation to the very low renin levels, and frequently a failure of aldosterone production to rise even when renin is stimulated.

Hypokalemia occurs frequently in the low-renin hypertensives, especially in patients with high aldosterone output taking a high-sodium diet. Potassium depletion generally tends to increase PRA and to lower aldosterone output (13,14); but in the low renin patients, a low serum potassium concentration is evidently ineffective in stimulating renin release.

On a high-sodium intake, aldosterone secretion rate is high in patients with Conn's syndrome due to an adrenal adenoma or to bilateral adrenal hyperplasia, versus the ordinary hypertensive level of aldosterone excretion present in the remainder of the low-renin hypertensives and in other hypertensive patients on a high-sodium intake. The low-renin hypertensives have been divided into those with aldosterone excretion suppressible by salt loading to less than 12 μg per day, and those whose aldosterone excretion rate persists in excess of 12 μg, who are considered instances of "hyperaldosteronism". In the first group, characterized as patients with low renin and low-normal aldosterone, there were 12 cases. The patients with hyperaldosteronism consisted of 14 cases, of whom 4 have proven adenoma, 3 "probable adenoma", and 4 cases bilateral adrenal hyperplasia. The differential diagnosis was based on surgical findings in 5 cases, and on adrenal venograms and analysis of blood drawn from left and right adrenal veins in the remainder.

I will show you the results of sodium loading and sodium
deprivation in different hypertensive groups. Figure 1 shows the
urine aldosterone excretion in micrograms per day on 3 days of very
heavy sodium intake, followed by 6 days on the 10 mEq sodium diet.
Each point is the average of measurements in 12 to 26 cases in a
particular group. On the high-sodium intake, the abnormally sustained aldosterone excretion of the hypertensive patients contrasts
with the marked suppression of aldosterone excretion in normotensive
controls. All of the hypertensive groups on the high sodium intake
show a significant elevation above the normotensive controls. The
average aldosterone excretion of hypertensive cases with normal PRA
is indicated by the squares; with low-renin, normal-aldosterone by
open triangles pointing downward; with high-renin by the triangles
pointing upward; with hypertension induced by estrogen-containing
oral contraceptives, by the half-closed circles. The solid triangles
far above the average range represent low-renin hypertensives with
hyperaldosteronism due to adenoma or hyperplasia.

Now let us observe how the low-sodium diet influences the
aldosterone excretion rate. Normal controls show a steady rise in
aldosterone excretion, increasing through the six days of sodium
deprivation to a final level near 80 µg/day. The normal and high-
renin hypertensives resemble the normotensive controls during the
low sodium period. An exaggerated rise in PRA occurs during sodium
depletion in patients taking oral contraceptives. I would like to
draw your attention particularly to the findings in the patients
with hyperaldosteronism, who show almost no change in aldosterone
excretion over this very wide range of sodium intake. Of equal
interest is the low-renin group who excrete normal quantities of
aldosterone on a high-sodium diet; they fail to increase aldosterone
production during sodium deprivation. Their aldosterone levels on
the fourth and fifth days of the low sodium diet are significantly
lower than the aldosterone excretion of any other group.

Figure 2 shows the effect of the change in sodium intake on
the urinary excretion of sodium. On the high sodium intake, all
groups of normotensive controls and hypertensives excreted the
sodium load promptly and efficiently. Recalling the wide variation
in aldosterone secretion and excretion in the several groups, one
must infer that wide variations in aldosterone secretion do not
measurably influence the excretion of a continuous sodium load.

Sodium excretion is similar in all hypertensive groups during
the first three days of sodium deprivation, confirming the observations of Jerums and Doyle (10). After the fourth day of the low
sodium diet, a significant difference appears between the several
groups. The normotensive controls come into sodium balance by the
fifth day and urinary sodium falls again on the sixth day. The
hypertensive patients with normal or high renin show somewhat

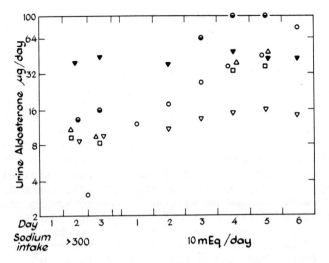

Figure 1.   Aldosterone excretion rate in normal controls (open
circles) and 5 groups of hypertensive patients with
different renin levels (see text for symbols) on
high and low-sodium diets.

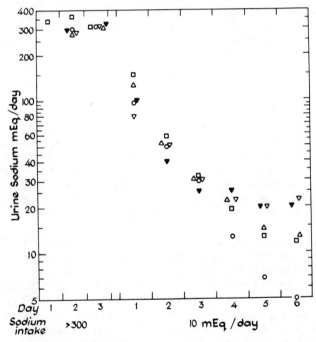

Figure 2.   Sodium excretion of normal controls and various
groups of hypertensive patients on high and low-
sodium diets.

higher urinary excretions of sodium, approaching balance by the 6th or 7th day. The highest urinary sodium excretion was observed in the low-renin cases.

A curious divergence between sodium excretion and aldosterone production appears in the low-renin hypertensives. Recall that the cases with hyperaldosteronism and low renin were within normal limits of aldosterone production on the low sodium diet, while the low renin, low-normal aldosterone group fell well below the other groups in aldosterone excretion. While we might attribute the slow and inadequate approach to sodium balance in the latter group to deficient aldosterone production, this explanation could scarcely apply in the patients with hyperaldosteronism. It must, therefore, be admitted that continued sodium wasting in the low-renin cases cannot be attributed entirely to deficient aldosterone production. Both of these groups with low renin start at a higher extracellular fluid volume and total body sodium than the other groups. We must inquire, therefore, whether the failure to diminish urinary sodium excretion in normal fashion is dependent on volume expansion or on low plasma renin.

Figure 3 shows the effect of changing sodium intake on urinary potassium excretion. Serum potassium is below normal in most patients with hyperaldosteronism, particularly in those with adrenal adenoma and very high aldosterone secretion. Patients with hyperaldosteronism show unusual losses of potassium during the period of sodium loading. The high urinary potassium excretion in hyperaldosteronism could accentuate low PRA if the predominant physiological stimulus is a high urine potassium rather than a low serum potassium. In most published experiments, serum and urine potassium move in the same direction, either downward in states of depletion, or toward higher levels after potassium loading (13,14). The interesting feature of the sodium-loaded patient with hyperaldosteronism is the opposite direction taken by urinary potassium (rising) and serum potassium (falling). The idea that there might be an area in the renal tubule which is sensitive to urinary potassium would, of course, require direct experimental confirmation, which might come from work such as Davis (15) has recently reported.

When placed on a low-sodium diet, the patients with hyperaldosteronism have the lowest potassium excretion rates, accompanied by a rise in serum potassium concentration. Plasma renin concentration increases appreciably, but the final level is sub-normal. In the low-renin cases without hyperaldosteronism, serum and urinary potassium occupy a position intermediate between the cases with hyperaldosteronism and the essentially normal findings in the hypertensive patients with normal PRA and aldosterone.

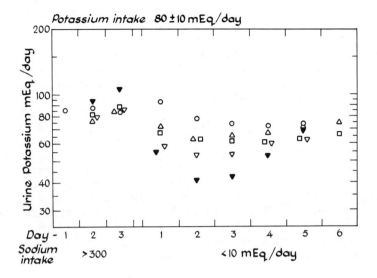

Figure 3. Potassium excretion of normal controls and various
           groups of hypertensive patients on high and low-
           sodium diets.

     Summarizing these findings, there are some interesting and
unexpected similarities between the low-renin group with hyperaldosteronism and other low-renin cases with ordinary aldosterone
production which does not rise normally during sodium deprivation.
Both of these groups have a subnormal plasma renin which does not
rise normally during sodium deprivation. Both low-renin groups have
a flat aldosterone response to the low-sodium diet, albeit at very
different levels. Both low-renin groups tend to lose sodium on the
low-sodium regime to approximately the same extent despite the wide
differences in aldosterone levels. All of the low-renin cases
start with higher extracellular volume and show a greater loss of
weight and exchangeable sodium during sodium depletion. Although
the low-renin cases lose more sodium and weight than the other
groups, ending at about the same extracellular volume as the other
hypertensive patients, the deficiency in plasma renin activity
persists on the low-sodium regime, and PRA shows less increase under
the stimulus of posture.

     What common factors are responsible for the similarities bet-
ween the low-renin cases with hyperaldosteronism and those with
normal or low aldosterone levels? In terms of etiology, it seems
unlikely that all of the cases with low plasma renin activity will
eventually turn out to have hyperaldosteronism, but it must be
admitted that a few patients emerge as clear-cut instances of

hyperaldosteronism under continued observation over a period of a
year or more. Only two of the 16 low-renin cases whose aldosterone
was initially suppressible have subsequently developed high, non-
suppressible aldosterone levels. Possibly additional cases may
emerge, but we doubt that all of the low-renin cases represent
instances of occult hyperaldosteronism. We would propose that there
are a number of features common to all the low-renin cases. There
appears to be a consistent expansion of extracellular fluid volume.
This may be related to a high-sodium intake and may have some possible connection with the non-suppressible aldosterone production, or
other adrenal steroid secretion. The expansion of exchangeable
sodium is accompanied by a slackness in the sodium-retaining control
system, which fails to respond properly and effectively to sodium
deprivation, even though extracellular volume and exchangeable
sodium reach a level sufficient to evoke normal responses in the
other cases. A similar blunting of the expected responses has been
seen after removal of an aldosterone-producing adenoma, when some
time must elapse before PRA increases normally.

It is interesting to speculate on the implications of continuing sodium loss in the low-renin cases. We suspect that this loss
originates in the proximal renal tubule, which rejects a larger
fraction of filtered sodium in the patient with high extracellular
volume. Increased tubular sodium reaching the macula densa would
tend to suppress renin release. Urinary potassium loss occurs only
if aldosterone is very high and non-suppressible by high-sodium
intake. On the low-sodium diet, the low-renin patient retains
significant amounts of potassium only if he is K-depleted, while a
small sodium loss persists regardless of the aldosterone level.
Observations, which suggest continuing proximal tubular rejection
of sodium, are the persistent sodium loss regardless of aldosterone
level, and the failure of renin to rise on the low-sodium diet.

We have also considered the possible effect of chronic extracellular volume expansion on the autonomic nervous system. Blunting
of renin response to physiological stimuli has been reported after
renal denervation (16,17). Collins (18) has found a significant
rise in urinary norepinephrine when normotensive and hypertensive
patients first stand in the morning. This rise is enhanced when the
patient has been on a low-sodium diet. Low-renin hypertensives
have a subnormal increase in norepinephrine under these conditions.
Other observers (7) have not found a significant difference in 24-
hour catecholamine excretion between low-renin and other hypertensive
cases. For the time being, we can only say that the failure of
renin to rise after standing can be correlated with reduced catecholamine excretion in the low-renin cases.

While final interpretation of all these findings will require
further study, it seems reasonable to relate the suppression of
renin in hypertension to chronic extracellular fluid volume expansion.

In some cases, excessive aldosterone production is primary, but
the cause of sodium retention in the majority of low-renin hypertensives remains to be described. Abnormalities of potassium
metabolism, which are most prominent in patients with hyperaldosteronism, but which also occur in low-renin hypertensives without
hyperaldosteronism, must also be considered as possible factors in
suppressed PRA. Decreased catecholamine release can be correlated
with the subnormal postural response of PRA in the low-renin
hypertensives.

ACKNOWLEDGMENTS

This research was supported by Research and Training Grants
from the National Institute of Arthritis and Metabolic Diseases
(AM-03062 and AM-5021). Dr. Luetscher received a Research Career
Award (AM-14176). Dr. Beckerhoff was a Fellow of the Bay Area
Heart Research Committee.

Data analyzed in this report were collected from patients
under the care of Drs. Myron H. Weinberger, R. Dennis Collins and
Robert Wilkinson. Anne Dowdy, Carol Gonzales, George Nokes and
Irene Beckerhoff contributed expert laboratory assistance. Dr.
A. Ganguly and Sandra Karsen helped with computer programming and
statistical analyses. The authors thank the staff of the General
Clinical Research Center (FR-70) and Stanford University Advanced
Computer for Medical Research (ACME FR-311).

REFERENCES

1.   Laragh, J.H., J.E. Sealey and S.C. Sommers, Patterns of
        Adrenal Secretion and Urinary Excretion of Aldosterone and
        Plasma Renin Activity in Normal and Hypertensive Subjects.
        Circulation Res. 18-19 (Suppl I): 158, 1966.
2.   Kirkendall, W.M., A. Fitz and M.L. Armstrong, Symposium on
        Hypertension: Hypokalemia and the Diagnosis of Hypertension.
        Dis. Chest 45: 337, 1964.
3.   De Champlain, J., J. Genest, R. Veyrat, et al., Factors
        controlling Renin in Man. Trans. Ass. Am. Physicians, 78:
        135, 1965.
4.   Brown, J.J., D.L. Davies, R. Fraser et al., Plasma Electrolytes,
        Renin and Aldosterone in the Diagnosis of Primary Hyper-
        aldosteronism. Lancet 2: 55, 1968.
5.   Conn, J.W., D.R. Rovner and E.L. Cohen, Normal and Altered
        Function of the Renin-Angiotensin-Aldosterone System in
        Man: Applications in Clinical and Research Medicine. Ann.
        Int. Med. 63: 266, 1965.
6.   Helmer, O.H., The Renin-Angiotensin System and its Relation to
        Hypertension. Prog. Cardiovas. Dis. 8: 117, 1965.

7.   Jose, A., J.R. Crout, N.M. Kaplan, Suppressed Plasma Renin
     Activity in Hypertension. Ann. Int. Med. 72:9, 1970.
8.   Weinberger, M.H., A.J. Dowdy, G.W. Nokes and J.A. Luetscher,
     Plasma Renin Activity and Aldosterone Secretion in Hyper-
     tensive Patients during High and Low Sodium Intake and
     Administration of Diuretic. J. Clin. Endocr. 28: 359, 1968.
9.   Kuchel, O., L.M. Fishman, G.W. Liddle et al., Effect of
     Diazoxide on Plasma Renin Activity in Hypertensive Patients.
     Ann. Int. Med. 67: 791, 1967.
10. Jerums, G. and A.E. Doyle, Renal Sodium Handling and Responsive-
     ness of Plasma Renin Levels in Hypertension. Clin. Sci.
     37: 79, 1969.
11. Woods, J.W., G.W. Liddle, B.G. Stant, Jr. et al., Effect of an
     Adrenal Inhibitor in Hypertensive Patients with Suppressed
     Renin. Arch. Int. Med. (Chicago), 123: 366, 1969.
12. Collins, R.D., M.H. Weinberger, A.J. Dowdy, G.W. Nokes,
     C.M. Gonzales and J.A. Luetscher, Abnormally Sustained
     Aldosterone Secretion during Salt Loading in Patients with
     various forms of Benign Hypertension. Relation to Plasma
     Renin Activity. J. Clin. Invest. 49: 1415, 1970.
13. Veyrat, R., H.R. Brunner, E.L. Manning and A.F. Muller, Inhibi-
     tion of Plasma Renin Activity by Potassium. J. Urol. Nephrol.
     73: 271, 1967.
14. Brunner, H.R., L. Baer, J.E. Sealey, J.G.G. Ledingham and
     J.H. Laragh, The Influence of Potassium Administration and
     Potassium Deprivation on Plasma Renin in Normal and Hyper-
     tensive Subjects. J. Clin. Invest. 49: 2128, 1970.
15. Blaine, E.H., J.O. Davis and R.T. Witty, Renin Release after
     Hemorrhage and after Suprarenal Aortic Constriction in
     Dogs without Sodium Delivery to the Macula Densa.
     Circulation Res. 27: 1081, 1970.
16. Bunag, R.D., I.H. Page and J.W. McCubbin, Neural Stimulation
     of Renin Release. Circulation Res. 19: 851, 1966.
17. Vander, A.J., Control of Renin Secretion. Physiol. Rev. 47:
     359, 1967.
18. Collins, R.D., M.H. Weinberger, C. Gonzales, G.W. Nokes and
     J.A. Luetscher, Catecholamine Excretion in Low Renin
     Hypertension. Clin. Res. 18: 167, 1970.

MECHANISMS OF SODIUM RETENTION IN CONGESTIVE HEART FAILURE

C.R. Ayers, R.E. Bowden and J.P. Schrank

Department of Internal Medicine, Division of Cardiology

University of Virginia, Charlottesville, Virginia

INTRODUCTION

The mechanisms involved in sodium and water retention in congestive heart failure have not been clearly delineated. It has been shown by many observers that the renal blood flow and glomerular filtration rate are decreased in congestive heart failure. The GFR is better preserved than the renal blood flow, thus an increase in filtration fraction (1-4). The role of aldosterone in sodium retention in congestive heart failure is not clear. The plasma renin activity and aldosterone secretion and excretion rates are variable and not always increased even though sodium retention from the urine is nearly complete (5-8).

A mechanism, other than the aldosterone secretion rate, that can lead to an elevated concentration of aldosterone in the plasma is the rate of clearance of aldosterone from the blood. Normally more than 95% of the aldosterone is metabolized or conjugated with one circulation through the liver (9-12). It has been shown that the metabolic clearance rate of aldosterone is reduced in congestive heart failure and that this may be due to a decrease in liver blood flow or a decrease in extraction by the liver (7,9,12).

The present work was performed to evaluate the relative importance of plasma renin activity, aldosterone secretion rate, metabolic clearance rate and renal function in sodium retention in patients with congestive heart failure and the effects of exercise on plasma renin activity and aldosterone metabolism.

MATERIALS AND METHODS

Patients. The subjects for study were selected from the general hospital population and divided into three groups. Group I consisted of 7 patients with mild heart disease who had never developed pulmonary edema or signs of peripheral congestion of the circulation. Six patients were maintained on a 110 mEq sodium diet (one of this group became short of breath on this sodium intake and was given a 60 mEq diet.) All patients maintained nearly a constant body weight during the study. Group II included 8 patients with severe heart disease and congestion of the circulation. All patients had some form of myocardial disease except one (#7), who had constrictive pericarditis. All of these patients were retaining sodium and water at rest. Therapy consisted of digoxin, low sodium diet and diuretics. These patients were admitted to the Clinical Research Center and all but one were maintained on a 30 mEq sodium diet. Digoxin was continued but diuretics were withheld. All patients in this group gained weight on this diet except one patient (#7), whose diet was then increased to 60 mEq per day. This sodium intake increased his body weight by 2.4 kilograms during the 7 days of the study. All patients in this group were grossly edematous and had jugular venous distention, hepatic enlargement, ascites and pretibial edema. Group III represents 5 patients with symptomatic mitral stenosis but without evidence of peripheral venous congestion and edema at the time of study. Four of the 5 patients received cardiac catheterization and were found to have moderate to severe increase in the gradient across the mitral valve and increased pulmonary artery pressure. One patient refused catheterization. He had physical and x-ray evidence of significant mitral stenosis with pulmonary hypertension. All of these patients were maintained on a 110 mEq sodium diet and none increased body weight or exhibited a positive sodium balance.

All three groups of patients studied received 80 mEq of potassium per day. The patients were admitted to the Clinical Research Center and started on controlled sodium intake. They were allowed bathroom privileges but were otherwise in bed or sitting in an armchair. After 3 days equilibration period the study was begun. They remained in bed for the supine part of the aldosterone disappearance study. Blood was withdrawn for plasma renin activity. Ten microcuries of 1,2 H^3-aldosterone (New England Nuclear Company) was diluted to 50 cc in saline. A 1 cc aliquot was taken for counting and to check for radiochemical purity of aldosterone in two chromatographic systems. The remainder was given intravenously to the patient. Twenty milliliter blood samples were withdrawn at 1, 3, 5, 10, 15, 30, 45 and 60 minute intervals. A 24 hour urine sample was collected to measure the aldosterone secretion rate, creatinine clearance, and sodium and potassium excretion. On the second day of study the patient's maximum exercise tolerance was determined. After

15 minutes of exercise, 10 µc of 1,2 H³-aldosterone was given intravenously and blood samples were withdrawn at the above time intervals. The patients continued to exercise throughout the 60 minute
period of the disappearance curve. With the exception of one patient, Group I exercised on a treadmill at 1.7 mph at 5°. One patient, because of foot drop, exercised during the test at 20 kpm/
hour on a bicycle ergometer. Six patients in Group II, because of
shortness of breath, could only walk slowly on the floor. Patients
#3 and #7 were able to ride the bicycle at 20 kpm/hour during the
test. In Group III patients #1 and #2 were able to walk on the
treadmill during the exercise portion of the test at 1.7 mph. Patients #3 and #4 could only walk on the floor. Patient #5 rode the
bicycle ergometer at 20 kpm/hour during the exercise test period.

To determine the ability of the liver to metabolize aldosterone
an oral dose of 10 µc 1,2 H³-aldosterone was given to each patient
and the appearance of unmetabolized, unconjugated 1,2 H³-aldosterone
in the plasma was determined. Blood samples were withdrawn at 10,
20, 30 and 40 minutes to determine the peak 1,2 H³-aldosterone
counts.

A separate 24 hour urine was collected in acid for determination of urinary excretion of norepinephrine.

Aldosterone Secretion Rate. The aldosterone secretion rate
was determined using the method of Ulich and Laragh (13). The
sample was hydrolyzed at pH 1 for 12 hours and then extracted with
ethyl diacetate and evaporated. The aldosterone was then separated
from its metabolites by chromatographing the sample in four systems.
(1) Mobile phase - toluene, stationary phase - 22% propylene glycol
in acetone. The sample was then acetylated with C^{14} acetic anhydride of known specific activity after the first chromatography.
(2) Mobile phase - 50% methylcyclohexane and toluene, stationary
phase - 56% formamide in methanol. (3) Mesitylene: methanol: water
(300:200:100). (4) Celite column - isooctane: methylene chloride:
methanol: water (1500:450:600:100). The fraction containing the
aldosterone was then counted simultaneously for H^3 and C^{14} and the
secretion rate calculated using the standard equation.

Plasma Aldosterone. The 1,2 H³-aldosterone was separated from
its metabolites by using the above first three chromatographic
systems. C^{14}-aldosterone (500 cpm) was added to 10 ml plasma to
correct for losses in the procedure. Cold aldosterone (100 µgm)
was added for chromatographic marker. The aldosterone was then
extracted from the plasma with 10 volumes methylene chloride, dried
and chromatographed in System 1. The spot was identified under
ultraviolet light and eluted from the paper with methanol. The
sample was then dried and acetylated with "cold" acetic anhydride
in the presence of pyridine. The aldosterone diacetate was then
chromatographed in Systems 2 and 3. The sample was then eluted,

dried and the H^3 and C^{14} were counted simultaneously in a scintillation counter. The loss of C^{14} in the procedure was determined
and the 1,2 H^3-aldosterone counts were corrected for losses in the
procedure. The H^3/C^{14} ratios were calculated after each chromatographic system. The ratios were nearly constant after the second
system. In addition 10 samples were chromatographed in a Bush 5
system and rerun in System 2 without a significant change in the
H^3/C^{14} ratio. The corrected 1,2 H^3-aldosterone counts were then
plotted semi-logarithmically against time.

The least squares fit method was used to best fit the data
(14-17). A two exponential model was used. The volumes of distribution, half-life, metabolic clearance rate were computed using
methods previously described (16-19).

The plasma renin activity was measured by a rat bioassay
method using a modification of Pickens' method (20). EDTA was
used as the anticoagulant; DFP was added to the plasma and the
sample was incubated at pH 5.5 for 16 and 24 hours and then frozen.
The sample was then assayed against synthetic angiotensin II in a
pentolinium-treated rat using the standard 4 point assay method.

Informed written consent was obtained from each patient
participating in the study. The research proposal was approved
by the University of Virginia School of Medicine Committee on
Human Experimentation.

RESULTS

The plasma renin activity in the 3 groups of patients is
tabulated in Table I. The supine renin activity is not significantly different in Group I (mild heart disease) and Group II (severe
heart disease). The supine values in these two groups are not
different from the supine value of 1.2 ± 0.5 in normal subjects
taking a 110 mEq sodium diet. Group I did not have a significant
rise in renin activity with 75 minutes of exercise, the rise in
Group II was significantly elevated with far less work stimulus
than Group I. The supine plasma renin in the mitral stenosis
group was greatly increased in one patient even though she was not
retaining sodium at the time of study. This group of patients
increased their plasma renin activity with exercise more readily
than either Group I or Group II; a very large increment of increase
in plasma renin activity was noted in two of the patients. The
aldosterone secretion rates have been completed in 10 patients
(Table II). The four patients studied in Group II (severe heart
disease) did not differ significantly from Group I (mild heart
disease).

TABLE I

Plasma Renin Activity

Patient	Group I Supine	Group I Exercise	Group II Supine	Group II Exercise	Group III Supine	Group III Exercise
1	1.2*	1.8	0.8	1.2	3.4	5.0
2	3.0	1.3	2.6	2.8	2.6	5.9
3	1.4	2.0	2.2	3.8	28.6	88.1
4	2.0	3.2	0.7	1.1	1.3	2.5
5	1.3	1.8	0.9	4.3	4.2	35.8
6	0.2	1.1	0.4	9.2		
7	0.5	0.9	0.6	4.2		
8			0.6	0.7		
Mean ±S.E.	1.4 ±.4 $P<.4$	1.7 ±.3	1.1 ±.3 $P<.01$	3.4 ±1.0	8.0 ±1.0 $P<.2$	27.5 ±5.2

* millimicrograms angiotensin II/ml/hr of incubation

TABLE II

Aldosterone Secretion Rate

μgm/24 hrs.

Patient	Group I	Group II	Group III
1	89	105	46
2	141	85	40
3	235	61	
4	204	123	
Mean ±S.E.	167 ±32	94 ±13	43

Difference in Group I and Group II is not significant.

The volume of distribution, half-life of the slow component of the disappearance curve and the metabolic clearance rate of aldosterone supine and during exercise are tabulated for Group I in Table III, Group II in Table IV and Group III in Table V. The volume of distribution (V_1) for the first exponential of the disappearance curve (most rapid declining phase of the disappearance curve) does not differ significantly in the three groups, neither in the supine position nor during exercise. The volume of distribution (V_2) of the second exponential (the slow declining phase of the curve) is significantly less (p < 0.01) in Group II, which had marked edema, than in either Group I or Group III which were edema free. This decreased volume of distribution did not change with exercise. Exercise did not alter the (V_2) volume of distribution in either Group I or Group III.

The mean supine half-life (T 1/2) of the second component of the disappearance curve in Group I was 38.1 ± 6.1 Two of the patients' values were higher than normal values reported by other workers. The T 1/2 did not change in this group with exercise; all the values are within normal limits reported by other observers. The metabolic clearance rate (liters/24 hours) was 1226 ± 194 L/24 hours in the supine position, which corresponds to normal values of other investigators (7,9,11,12,19), and did not change significantly during exercise. The T 1/2 of the slow component of the supine disappearance curves in Group II (salt retaining group) did not differ significantly from Group I; however, there was significant prolongation of the half-life with exercise (p < 0.02). The metabolic clearance rate in Group II was significantly less (p < 0.02) than in Group I and a further decrease from 588 ± 84 to 425 ± 22 L/day occurred during mild exercise (p < .01). The T 1/2 in Group III was normal in the supine position but increased in all five patients with exercise (p < 0.02). The metabolic clearance rate decreased from 1957 ± 1000 to 830 ± 329 L/day during the exercise period (p < 0.05)

The liver function tests performed in Group II are tabulated in Table VI. The bilirubin was elevated in 5 of the 8 patients (one patient, #2, was subsequently proven to have a pulmonary embolus). The SGOT, LDH and alkaline phosphatase were elevated in three patients. Six of the 8 patients did not completely metabolize the ingested H^3-aldosterone. A detectable quantity of unmetabolized, unconjugated 1,2 H^3-aldosterone appeared in the plasma of these 6 patients. Patient #2 had a large quantity traverse the liver unmetabolized. The peak 1,2 H^3-aldosterone in the extra-cellular fluid could have equalled as much as 20-30% of the ingested dose. None of Group I or Group III had abnormal liver function tests and there was no detectable 1,2 H^3-aldosterone in the plasma after ingestion of 10 µc of tritiated aldosterone.

TABLE III

Metabolism of 1,2 H^3-Aldosterone

Group I

Patient		V_1	V_2	T 1/2	MCR	V_1	V_2	T 1/2	MCR
		Supine				Exercise			
R.D.	1	2.4	19.4	27.2	1130	2.7	23.6	22.7	1114
J.L.	2	1.9	11.6	34.7	617	1.8	11.5	25.7	737
W.V.	3	6.3	32.4	26.7	1951	6.0	34.3	26.0	1975
V.S.	4	4.6	30.6	56.8	870	1.8	10.0	22.5	687
E.M.	5	2.1	24.2	39.4	1312	1.4	13.4	34.4	899
M.L.	6	7.3	37.7	62.9	848	10.6	20.5	28.0	1258
E.M.B.	7	1.0	16.5	19.3	1856	7.5	25.2	39.6	1249
Mean		3.6	24.6	38.1	1226	4.5	19.8	28.4	1131
± S.E.		±0.9	±3.6	±6.1	±194	±1.3	±3.3	±2.4	±165

V_1 = volume of distribution of the first exponential (rapid declining phase) of the H^3-aldosterone disappearance curve.

V_2 = volume of distribution of the second exponential of the H^3-aldosterone disappearance curve (slow component of the curve).

T 1/2 = half-life of the second exponential of the H^3-aldosterone disappearance curve.

MCR = metabolic clearance rate in liters/24 hours.

Supine and exercise differences are not significantly different.

TABLE IV

Metabolism of Aldosterone

Group II

Patient		V_1	V_2	T 1/2	MCR	V_1	V_2	T 1/2	MCR
		Supine				Exercise			
J.J.	1	4.4	9.7	34	454	1.3	12.7	40	434
A.T.	2	1.4	3.4	57	221	2.7	10.5	51	324
G.P.	3	19.2	7.3	41	679	20.2	5.2	55	389
A.J.	4	2.1	15.1	34	693	2.3	16.1	53	493
C.C.	5	6.2	6.6	40	566	5.4	6.4	53	432
H.M.	6	3.0	18.6	27	940	3.4	15.1	49	482
S.T.	7	2.8	18.4	51	565	2.4	20.7	69	423
Mean		5.6	11.3	40.6	588	5.4	12.4	52.9	425
± S.E.		±2.3	±2.4	±3.9	±84	±2.5	±2.4	±3.3	±22
			p<.01					p<.02	p<.01

V_1 = volume of distribution of the first exponential (rapid declining phase) of the aldosterone disappearance curve.

V_2 = volume of distribution of the second exponential of the H^3-aldosterone disappearance curve (slow component of the curve).

T 1/2 = half-life of the second exponential of the H^3-aldosterone disappearance curve.

MCR = metabolic clearance rate.

Exercise T 1/2 and MCR are significantly changed from supine values. V_2 of Group II is significantly less than V_2 of Group I.

TABLE V

Metabolism of Aldosterone

Group III

Patient		V_1	V_2	Supine T 1/2	MCR	V_1	V_2	Exercise T 1/2	MCR
R.S.	1	16.7	17.4	41	1082	3.4	19.0	66	363
R.P.	2	2.9	25.6	44	1257	4.3	24.2	49	863
A.R.	3	3.6	16.8	34	908	11.7	34.6	212	246
T.H.	4	1.6	12.4	16	603	1.3	12.0	38	308
L.J.	5	40.5	18.9	10	5934	4.2	20.5	20	2371
Mean		13.1	18.2	29.0	1957	4.9	22.1	77	830
± S.E.		±7.4	±2.1	±6.8	±1000	±1.8	±3.7	±35	±329
								p<.02	p<.05

V_1 = volume of distribution of the first exponential (rapid declining phase) of the aldosterone disappearance curve.

V_2 = volume of distribution of the second exponential of the H^3-aldosterone disappearance curve (slow component of the curve).

T 1/2 - half-life of the second exponential of the H^3-aldosterone disappearance curve.

MCR = metabolic clearance rate.

The exercise T 1/2 and MCR are significantly different from the supine values.

TABLE VI

Liver Function Studies

Group II

Patients	Bilirubin[1] (mg%)	SGOT[2]	LDH[3]	ALK[4]	ABSORPTION[5] H^3-Aldosterone (% Ingested Dose/L)
1	0.8	26	74	2.8	0.03
2	3.2	66	146	8.8	0.72
3	2.3	40	44	7.0	0.16
4	1.8	40	115	4.3	0.14
5	0.6	41	81	4.5	0
6	0.9	32	84	4.2	0
7	3.5	95	375	13.3	0.64
8	2.5	75	160	6.0	0.14
Mean	1.95	52	135	6.0	0.21

[1] Total bilirubin in mg%. Normal range is 0.3 - 1.5 mg%.

[2] Serum glutamicoxaloacetic transaminase in international units. Normal range is up to 40 units.

[3] Lactic acid dehydrogenase in international units. Normal range is up to 120 units.

[4] Alkaline phosphatase. Normal range is up to 6 Bodansky units.

[5] Absorption of H^3-aldosterone in % ingested dose/L. Normal is 0.

The mean plasma concentration of aldosterone was calculated in 4 patients in Group I and Group II and tabulated in Table VII. The mean plasma concentration of 1.7 ± .4 µgm % in Group I did not differ significantly from the mean of 2.3 ± .6 µgm % in the 4 patients with marked edema in Group II.

The sodium excretion rate, renal function and norepinephrine excretion are shown in Table VIII. Sodium balance was present in Groups I and III at the time of study. There was sodium retention and weight gain in all patients in Group II. The clearance of creatinine from the plasma of patients in Group II with marked sodium retention and edema was significantly lower than the other two groups of patients without sodium retention and edema. One patient in Group I (#3) was discovered to have chronic parenchymal renal disease after the studies were underway.

The norepinephrine excretion in Group II was 77 ± 15 µgm/day. Four of the 8 patients exceeded the upper limit of normal for this laboratory (80 µgm/day). Group II norepinephrine excretion was significantly greater than either Group I or Group III (p < 0.01).

DISCUSSION

There are many factors known to influence sodium reabsorption by the kidney. The mechanisms most generally accepted are changes in the glomerular filtration rate, plasma aldosterone concentration, proximal peritubular hydrostatic (21) and oncotic pressure (22) and possibly a natriuretic hormone (23). All of these factors have been implicated in sodium and water retention in congestive heart failure but the relative importance of these factors has not been delineated.

The plasma concentration of aldosterone is determined by a number of factors. The present experiments show that aldosterone secretion rate may be normal while resting even though the patient may be retaining nearly all of the sodium from the urine and gaining weight. Other observers have also found that the secretion and excretion rates of aldosterone may be normal (5,7,8,9,12). The normal supine plasma renin activity in Group II (sodium retaining edematous group) also supports the view that increased aldosterone secretion is not necessary for nearly complete sodium retention in congestive heart failure. The patients with edema (Group II) had a larger increment of increase in the plasma renin activity with a much less "work stimulus" than Group I. Group III patients with mitral stenosis also tended to greatly increase plasma renin activity during exercise. This suggests that patients with significant heart disease are likely to have significantly greater aldosterone secretion rates with a given exercise stimulus than subjects

TABLE VII

Calculated Mean Resting Plasma Aldosterone Concentration

Patient	Group I			Group II		
	ASR	MCR	MPC	ASR	MCR	MPC
1	89	1130	0.8	104	453	2.3
2	141	617	2.3	85	221	3.9
3	235	1951	1.2	61	679	0.9
4	204	870	2.3	123	565	2.2
Mean	167	1142	1.7	93	479	2.3
± S.E.	±32	±289	±.4	±13	±98	±.6

ASR = aldosterone secretion rate (μgm/24 hours).

MCR = metabolic clearance rate of aldosterone (liters/24 hours).

MPC = mean plasma concentration of aldosterone (μgm/100 ml plasma).

The calculated mean plasma concentrations do not differ significantly in these two groups.

Table VIII

Sodium Excretion and Renal Function

Patient	Sodium Intake (mEq/day)	Sodium Excretion (mEq/day)	BUN (mg %)	CR (mg %)	Ccr (ml/min)	Norepinephrine Excretion (μgm/day)
Group I						
1	110	84	13	1.3	110	33
2	110	95	22	1.2	94	31
3	110	127	52	4.6	18	10
4	60*	54	26	1.0	124	20
5	110	90	14	1.2	92	12
6	110	108	28	1.9	88	10
7	110	71	13	1.3	94	9
Mean	103	90	24	1.7	89	18
± S.E.		±9	±5	±.4	±12	±4.2
Group II						
1	30	7	35	1.6	26	9
2	30	2	55	2.1	22	66
3	30	11	20	1.4	40	62
4	30	18	23	1.3	24	100
5	30	2	19	1.6	57	114
6	30	1	28	1.8	32	128
7	60*	34	17	1.4	98	110
8	30	12	55	2.9	20	27
Mean	34	11	32	1.8	40	77
±S.E.		±4	±6	±.06	±9	±15
					$p < .01$	$p < .01$
Group III						
1	110	65	14	1.4	77	28
2	110	74	15	1.4	82	16
3	110	103	18	0.9	74	51
4	110	100	19	1.3	33	20
5	110	74	17	1.2	95	16
Mean	110	82	17	1.2	72	26
±S.E.		±8	±1	±.09	±10	±7

BUN = blood urea nitrogen. Normal < 20 mg%.   Normal norepinephrine =
CR = creatinine. Normal 0.5 - 1.5 mg%.   < 80 μgm/24 hours
Ccr = clearance of creatinine.

with a normal cardiac reserve. It is also of interest that the supine plasma renin activity is normal in the patients with congestive heart failure even though marked renal vascular constriction is probably present.

The metabolic clearance rate of aldosterone from the plasma is also a factor in determining the plasma aldosterone concentration. The patients with minimal heart disease had normal values supine and did not change significantly during the period of moderate exercise. The Group II patients had a significantly decreased metabolic clearance rate while supine which is in accord with previous observations. The T 1/2 of the slow component of the disappearance curves of Group II was not significantly different from Group I in the supine position. The explanation for the decreased volume (V_2) of distribution is not apparent but has also been observed in dogs on a low sodium diet (17). The metabolic clearance rate decreased further in this group during exercise due to an increased half-life of aldosterone; the volume of distribution remained the same during exercise. The metabolic clearance rate in Group III with mitral stenosis was near normal in the supine position but decreased strikingly during exercise due to a decreased disappearance rate from the plasma. These findings suggest that this mechanism could increase the plasma aldosterone concentration significantly during exercise.

It has been shown that normally aldosterone is nearly 100% metabolized during one circulation through the liver and that about 90% of aldosterone is metabolized or conjugated by the liver (9,10, 11). These characteristics of aldosterone metabolism would make the plasma clearance essentially equal to the hepatic blood flow as long as the liver is nearly completely extracting and metabolizing aldosterone during one circulation through the liver. Previous observations have demonstrated that some patients with congestive heart failure do not completely metabolize aldosterone during one circulation (9). In the present experiments no measurable amount of unmetabolized or unconjugated orally administered H^3-aldosterone reached the peripheral blood except in the group with congestive heart failure, Group II. In only 2 of the 8 patients did a sizeable amount traverse the liver unmetabolized. This suggests that the hepatic blood flow is markedly decreased in Group II with congestive heart failure and that further reduction in flow occurs with the upright position and exercise. Marked changes in hepatic blood flow in congestive heart failure have been previously observed (24,25). The present work also suggests that the largest changes in hepatic flow occurred in the group with mitral stenosis. This group had near normal metabolic clearance rates supine but markedly decreased this with exercise suggesting marked redistribution of blood flow.

The 4 patients in Group II with measured aldosterone secretion rates have nearly the same calculated plasma aldosterone concentrations as the patients in Group I. This suggests that nearly complete sodium extraction from the glomerular filtrate can occur in the presence of a near normal plasma aldosterone concentration.

The creatinine clearance was reduced in Group II which is in accord with previous work. This is most likely due to marked reduction in renal blood flow (1-4). In three of the patients with marked sodium retention and edema formation Xenon[133] washout studies demonstrated a marked decrease in cortical blood flow. The greater increase in norepinephrine excretion in the edematous group suggests that the decrease in renal blood flow is mediated through the sympathetic nervous system. That the sympathetic nervous system is important in sodium conservation has been demonstrated by the previous natriuretic effect of sympatholytic agents (26). This stimulus is probably mediated through the baroreceptors (27).

The present findings suggest that almost complete sodium retention can occur in congestive heart failure with a normal plasma concentration of aldosterone and that probably the most important factor promoting sodium retention in heart failure is renal hemodynamic changes mediated by the sympathetic nervous system.

SUMMARY

The present data show that plasma renin activity and aldosterone secretion rate may be normal in patients with congestive heart failure and severe sodium retention. The metabolic clearance rate and the volume of distribution of aldosterone are decreased. The half-life of injected 1,2 H^3-aldosterone is normal in the supine position. There is an increase in plasma renin activity, decrease in metabolic clearance rate and prolongation of the half-life of aldosterone with exercise. The calculated plasma aldosterone concentration was normal in 4 of the patients with congestive heart failure.

The decreased creatinine clearance and the high excretion rate of catecholamines suggest that the sympathetic-nervous-system-induced renal hemodynamic changes are primarily responsible for renal retention of sodium. The hormonal changes are probably of secondary importance.

ACKNOWLEDGEMENTS

This work was supported by The Department of Internal Medicine, Division of Cardiology, University of Virginia, Charlottesville,

Virginia, The Virginia Heart Association, NIH Research Grant #RO1
HE 14066 and the Clinical Research Center, University of Virginia
Hospital, NIH Grant # RR00304.

REFERENCES

1.   Merrill, A.J., Edema and decreased renal blood flow in patients
      with chronic congestive heart failure: evidence of forward
      failure as the primary cause of edema. JCI. 25: 389, 1946.
2.   Bradley, S.E. and W.D. Blake, Pathogenesis of renal dysfunction
      during congestive heart failure. Am. J. Med. 6: 470, 1949.
3.   Mokotoff, R., G. Ross and L. Leiter, Renal plasma flow and
      sodium reabsorption and excretion in CHF. JCI. 27: 1, 1948.
4.   Bradley, S.E. and G.P. Bradley, Renal function during chronic
      anemia in man. Blood. 2: 192, 1947.
5.   Laragh, J.H., Hormones and the pathogenesis of congestive heart
      failure: vasopressin, aldosterone and angiotensin II.
      Circ. 25: 1015, 1962.
6.   Wolff, H.P., Aldosterone in congestive heart failure. Acta
      Cardiol. 20: 424, 1965.
7.   Camargo, C.A., A.J. Dowdy, E.W. Hancock et al., Decreased
      plasma clearance and hepatic extraction of aldosterone in
      patients with heart failure. JCI. 44: 356, 1965.
8.   Vecsei, P., G. Dusterdieck, J. Jahnecke et al., Secretion and
      turnover of aldosterone in various pathological states.
      Clin. Sci. 36: 241, 1969.
9.   Luetscher, J.A., C.A. Camargo, E.W. Hancock et al., Observations
      of aldosterone metabolism in congestive heart failure.
      Tr. A. Am. Phys. 77: 224, 1964.
10.   Bledsoe, T., G.W. Liddle, A. Riondel et al., Comparative fates
      of intravenously and orally administered aldosterone:
      evidence for extrahepatic formation of acid-hydrolyzable
      conjugate in man. JCI. 45: 264, 1966.
11.   Luetscher, J.A., E.W. Hancock, C.A. Camargo et al., Conjugation
      of $1,2-^3$H-aldosterone in human liver and kidneys and renal
      extraction of aldosterone and labeled conjugates from blood
      plasma. J. Clin. Endocr. 25: 628, 1965.
12.   Tait, J.F., J. Bougas, B. Little et al., Splanchnic extraction
      and clearance of aldosterone in subjects with minimal and
      marked cardiac dysfunction. J. Clin. Endocr. 25: 219, 1965.
13.   Ulich, S., J.H. Laragh and S. Lieberman, The isolation of a
      urinary metabolite of aldosterone and its use to measure the
      rate of secretion of aldosterone by the adrenal cortex of
      man. Tr. A. Am. Phys. 71: 225, 1958.
14.   Berman, M. and R. Schoenfeld, Invariants in experimental data
      in linear kinetics and the formulation of models. J. Appl.
      Phys. 27: 1361, 1956.
15.   Berman, M., E. Shahn and M. Weiss, The routine fitting of kin-
      etics data to models: a mathematical formation for digital
      computers. Biophys. J. 2: 275, 1962.

16. Ayers, C.R., J.O. Davis, S. Lieberman et al., The effects of chronic hepatic venous congestion on the metabolism of d-l-aldosterone and d-aldosterone. JCI. 41: 884, 1962.

17. Davis, J.O., M.J. Olichney, T.C. Brown et al., Metabolism of aldosterone in several experimental situations with altered aldosterone secretion. JCI. 44: 1433, 1965.

18. Tait, J.F., S.A.S. Tait, B. Little et al., The disappearance of 7-H^3-d-aldosterone in the plasma of normal subjects. JCI. 40: 72, 1961.

19. Tait, J.F., B. Little, S.A.S. Tait et al., The metabolic clearance rate of aldosterone in pregnant and nonpregnant subjects estimated by both single-injection and constant-infusion methods. JCI. 41: 2093, 1962.

20. Pickens, P.T., F.M. Bumpus, A.M. Lloyd et al., Measurement of renin activity in human plasma. Circulation Res. 17: 438, 1965.

21. Earley, L.E., J.A. Martino and R.M. Frudler, Factors affecting sodium reabsorption by the proximal tubule as determined during blockage of distal sodium reabsorption. JCI. 45: 1668, 1968.

22. Barry, M., K.H. Brenner, R.I. Falchuk et al., The relationship between peritubular capillary protein concentration and fluid reabsorption by the proximal tubule. JCI. 48: 1519, 1969.

23. Sealey, J.E., J.D. Kirshman and J.H. Laragh, Natriuretic activity in plasma and urine of salt-loaded man and sheep. JCI. 48: 2210, 1969.

24. Myers, J.D. and J.B. Hickam, An estimation of the hepatic blood flow and splanchnic oxygen consumption in heart failure. JCI. 27: 620, 1948.

25, Donald, K.W., Hemodynamics in chronic congestive heart failure. J. Chron. Dis. 9: 476, 1959.

26. Gill, J.R. Jr. and F.C. Bartter, Adrenergic nervous system in sodium metabolism. - II Effects of guanethidine on the renal response to sodium deprivation in normal man. New Eng. J. Med. 275: 1466, 1966.

27. Gilmore, J.P., Contribution of baroreceptors to the control of renal function. Circulation Res. 14: 301, 1964.

HYPERCALCIURIA AND INCREASED PLASMA RENIN ACTIVITY

W.J. Meyer III, S.A. Middler, C.S. Delea and F.C. Bartter

Endocrinology Branch, National Heart and Lung Institute

Bethesda, Maryland

INTRODUCTION

Among the patients with primary aldosteronism studied in this clinic, two were observed with hypercalciuria. A 46-year-old man with primary aldosteronism resulting from an adrenal adenoma was found to have nephrocalcinosis and hypercalciuria. A 57-year-old man with primary aldosteronism resulting from bilateral adrenal hyperplasia was found to have nephrolithiasis, osteoporosis and hypercalciuria. This suggested a relationship between aldosteronism on the one hand and hypercalciuria on the other and all subsequent patients with a history of hypercalciuria were examined for evidence of hyperaldosteronism. All patients showing serum potassium values below 3.5 mEq/L were further studied with respect to the renin-aldosterone system. Of 55 patients with hypercalciuria, 7 showed hypokalemia and were further studied. One of them had aldosteronism with suppressed plasma renin activity and at operation was shown to have adrenal hyperplasia. The present report concerns the findings in the other six patients.

MATERIALS AND METHODS

The presenting data on each patient are summarized in Table I. All of the patients studied had hypokalemia, some had hypertension and all had hypercalciuria. The diagnosis of renal tubular acidosis was ruled out by the presence in each patient of a urinary pH below 6 at a time when serum bicarbonate concentrations were normal.

245

TABLE I

Patient	Age (yrs)	Sex	Serum K (mEq/L)	B.P. (mmHg)	Urinary Ca (mg/day)	Nephro-calcinosis	Nephro-lithiasis
E.B.	48	F	3.4	150/110	297		
T.W.	47	M	3.4	150/100	168-212		x
D.B.	28	F	3.4	150/115	340	x	
N.R.	36	F	3.3	160/110	177-232	x	
W.G.	36	M	3.3	130/70	300	x	
J.M.	48	F	3.3	120/76	200-400		

All patients were studied on both 249 mEq and 9 mEq sodium
diets. The 9 mEq sodium diet was occasionally initiated with 2 ml
of Mercuhydrin. All diets were continued until the urinary sodium
equaled the intake; all high sodium intakes lasted at least 7 days.
All patients had both aldosterone secretion rates (ASR) and plasma
renin activities (PRA) measured on both regimens. The aldosterone
secretion rates were measured by injection of a known amount of
tritiated aldosterone and measurement of the specific activity of
aldosterone in a 24-hour urine. Plasma renin activity was measured
by a modification of Boucher's method in which bioassay pressor
effects are measured in a vagotomized pentolinium-treated rat (1).
PRA is expressed in ng% angiotensin II generated per 3 hours. Some
of the PRA's were measured as angiotensin I generated per ml of
plasma per hour as estimated by the radioimmunoassay method of
Haber (2). Normal values for the aldosterone secretion rates and
plasma renin activities on the various regimens are given in Table
II.

Case Reports:

E.B.   08-02-94
     This 48-year-old caucasian woman was first admitted in
December 1968 to the Clinical Center for evaluation of hyperparathyroidism. Her family history is positive for a parathyroid adenoma
in her daughter and hypertension in her mother. Her physical examination was remarkable for tender bones in her feet and legs,
diffuse thyroid enlargement, normal BP and multiple lipomata of the
skin. The following laboratory values were obtained during that
admission: Na, 141; K, 2.9; Cl, 107; and CO_2, 26 mEq/L; Ca, 11.9
and PO_4, 2.2 mg%; Mg, 1.74 mEq/L; alkaline phosphatase, 372 I.U.;
albumin, 3.8 g%; T-4, 3.6 ug%; RAI, 23.9% with an abnormal scan;
antithyroid antibody titer, 1:512; creatinine 0.5 mg%; urinary
calcium, 212 mg/d; multiple lytic lesions of the bone. During her
hospitalization she underwent a parathyroidectomy for parathyroid
adenoma. A thyroid biopsy showed chronic thyroiditis. After discharge she did well on dihydrotachysterol 0.5 mg/d with supplemental
calcium and potassium. On readmission in July 1969 it was noted
that her bones were healing. At that time she was first noted to
be hypertensive with a BP 160/100. Her laboratory values showed
the following: Na, 137; K, 3.7; Cl, 106; CO_2, 25 mEq/L; Ca, 8.9;
PO_4, 3.9 mg%; alkaline phosphatase, 33 I.U.; albumin, 4.2 g%; T-4,
5.7 ug%; a positive urine culture and a normal rapid sequence IVP.
She was discharged on the same medication and had an uneventful
course except for one recurrence of an urinary tract infection.

     Two weeks prior to her admission in August 1970 she discontin-
ued all medication. Her admission physical examination was remarkable for a BP of 228/125, a slightly firm nodular thyroid, one and
one-half times normal size and a movable, firm nontender breast mass.

Her laboratory values on this admission were the following: Na, 140;
K, 3.1; Cl, 108; and CO_2, 27 mEq/L; Ca, 9.9; and PO_4, 2.4 mg%;
alkaline phosphatase, 23 I.U.; albumin 4.2 g%; T-4, 3.9 ug%;
creatinine clearance, 90 ml/min; normal renal size; normal rapid
sequence IVP; urinary calcium, 340 mg/d; 17 hydroxycorticosteroids,
8.0 mg/d; VMA, 3.2 and 2.4 mg/d; a normal response to NH_4Cl load;
total body potassium 62.3 mEq/kg (28.7 - 46.0 normal). The results
of the renin-aldosterone studies are shown in Table II. Her blood
pressure was unchanged by sodium restriction. The patient refused
investigation of her breast mass. She was thought to have normal
parathyroid function and was discharged on only Gantrisin 6.0 g/d
for an urinary tract infection.

T.W. 04-63-71 (Figure 1)
     This 39-year-old caucasian man was admitted to the Clinical
Center for the first time in November 1962 with the chief complaint
of hypertension of at least 16 years' duration. In 1958 he developed
his first renal stone. His family history is unremarkable. Upon
admission in 1962 his physical examination was normal except for
a BP of 160/120. Other studies revealed the following: Na, 141;
K, 4.8; Cl, 106; and CO_2, 27 mEq/L; Ca, 11.7 and PO_4, 3.0 mg%;
albumin, 4.0 g%; metanephrines 0.43 mg/d; urinary calciums, 166 to
238 mg/d; normal renogram; normal rapid sequence IVP. After parathyroidectomy he was free of stones until 1970. The resultant
hypoparathyroidism has required therapy with vitamin D and supplemental calcium. At the time of admission in August 1970 his BP was
well-controlled with Aldomet, 500 mg/d, and spironolactone, 50 mg/d.
During the first month of his hospitalization serum potassium
concentrations below 3.5 were noted on several occasions in spite
of the rest of the electrolytes being normal. Other pertinent data
include the following: Ca, 9.7 and PO_4, 5.6 mg%; Mg, 1.55 mEq/L;
alkaline phosphatase, 47 I.U.; albumin, 3.6 g%; T-4, 5.9 ug%;
creatinine, 1.2 mg%; urinalysis: sp.gr. 1.020, pH, 5.5, negative for
protein, sugar and acetone; creatinine clearance, 104 ml/min; normal
rapid sequence IVP; urinary calcium excretion, 168 to 212 mg/d;
calcium absorption 36% (31-59% normal) (3). One and one-half months
after admission his renin and aldosterone system was studied (see
Table II). His hypertension was not affected by changes in sodium
intake. As an outpatient he has done well on Aldomet.

D.B. 08-63-94 (Figure 2)
     This 28-year-old caucasian woman was admitted to the Clinical
Center with the chief complaint of hypertension associated with
vertigo and lightheadedness. Her father and father's cousin have
nephrolithiasis. She had received no therapy for her hypertension
prior to her admission and had discontinued Enovid 21 just ten days
prior to admission and 30 days prior to the study of her renin-
aldosterone system. Her physical examination was normal except for

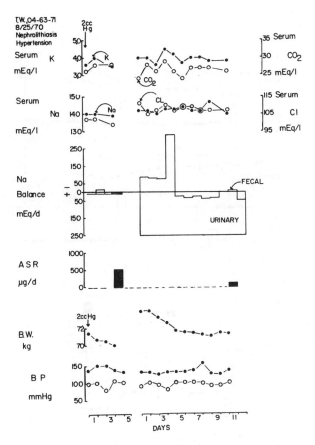

Figure 1. The effects of low and high sodium intakes on serum
potassium and carbon dioxide concentrations, serum
sodium and chloride concentrations, sodium balance,
aldosterone secretion rate, body weight and blood
pressure in patient T.W. with nephrolithiasis.

a BP of 170/120. Her initial studies showed the following: Na, 139;
K, 3.2; Cl, 102; and CO_2, 31 mEq/L; Ca, 9.4 and PO_4, 4.4 mg%;
Mg, 1.5 mEq/L; alkaline phosphatase, 32 I.U.; albumin, 4.3 g%;
creatinine, 0.8 and BUN, 12 mg%; urinalysis: sp. gr. 1.009, pH, 5.5,
negative for protein, sugar and acetone; creatinine clearance,
122 ml/min, normal renogram and renal scan, normal renal size with
nephrocalcinosis, normal rapid sequence IVP; urinary Ca, 333 mg and
355 mg/d; metanephrine, 0.45 mg/d; 17 hydroxycorticosteroids, 7.2 and
9.3 mg/d; Ca absorption, 44% (normal 31 to 59%) and total body potassium,47.7 mEq/kg (28.7 to 46.0, normal). Her renin-aldosterone system
was studied on metabolic balance. Her BP and hypercalciuria were
greatly improved on a low-sodium intake in the hospital. Her BP
has been well controlled as an outpatient on a low-sodium diet with

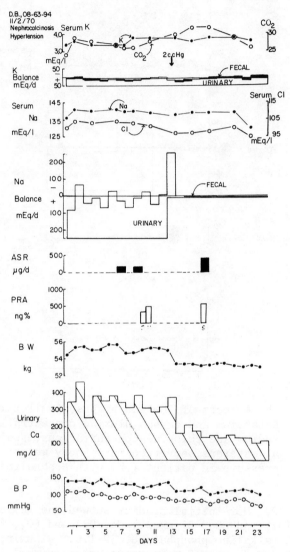

Figure 2.   The effects of high- and low-sodium intakes on serum
potassium and carbon dioxide concentrations, potassium
balance, serum sodium and chloride concentrations,
sodium balance, aldosterone secretion rates, plasma
renin activity, body weight, urinary calcium and blood
pressure in patient D.B. with nephrocalcinosis.

the administration of 50 mg Diuril and 100 mg triamterine each day.
Her hypertension recurred when her medication was discontinued
eight months later.

N.R.   00-06-09   (Figure 3)
     This 36-year-old caucasion woman was first referred to the
National Institutes of Health in 1965 because of myasthenia gravis
of two years'duration. Family history is remarkable in that her
mother has hypertension. At the time of her admission a normal BP
(100/65) and serum potassium concentration (4.5) were recorded.
In March 1966 her myasthenia became worse and she presented in the
emergency room with respiratory arrest. Her subsequent hospitalization was prolonged and included two tracheostomies and a thymec-
tomy. Her blood pressure during that hospitalization was recorded
as high as 130/90. In May of the same year her BP was 140/100 with
a normal serum potassium.

     In the spring of 1971 she was readmitted for evaluation.
During that admission her myasthenia was treated with 100 mg/d
ephedrine, 360 mg/d Mestinon, and 100 mg secobarbitol at bedtime
Her physical examination was remarkable for hypertension, BP 150/110,
and generalized muscle weakness with ptosis. During evaluation
for hypertension, nephrocalcinosis was found which, in retrospect,
was present on a 1968 film. Her laboratory values were the following: Na, 139; K, 3.3; Cl, 110; and CO_2, 27 mEq/L; Ca, 9.9; and PO_4
3.4 mg%; Mg, 1.8 mEq/L; alkaline phosphatase, 27 I.U.; albumin,
3.88g%; T-4, 3.5 ug%; creatinine, 0.8 mg%; urinalysis: sp.gr. 1.018,
pH 5.0; negative for protein, sugar and acetone; creatinine clearance 92 ml/min; normal renal size with bilateral nephrocalcinosis;
normal rapid sequence IVP; renogram showing no hypertensive renovascular disease; urinary calciums, 177 to 232 mg/d; VMA 1.4 mg/d;
5-OH indolacetic acids, 2.3 mg/d; 17-hydroxycorticosteroids, 3.2
mg/d; normal urinary aminoacids; Ca   absorption, 43% (31-59%
normal); total body potassium 50.9 (28.7 - 46.0 normal). Her renin-
aldosterone system was evaluated and the results are in Table II.
Her BP became normal on sodium restriction and she has been well-
controlled as an outpatient on that regime.

W.G.   07-96-04   (Figure 4)
     This 36-year-old caucasian man was first referred to the
National Institutes of Health in 1968 for treatment of his recurrent
nephrolithiasis and secondary hypoparathyroidism.
     He was well until age 25 when he began having kidney stones.
At that time he was found to have hypercalcemia and hypercalciuria.
A parathyroidectomy resulted in hypoparathyriodism which required
treatment with vitamin D and calcium supplementation. Since that
time he has continued to have multiple kidney stones. On several
occasions he has developed vitamin D intoxication with hypercalcemia.

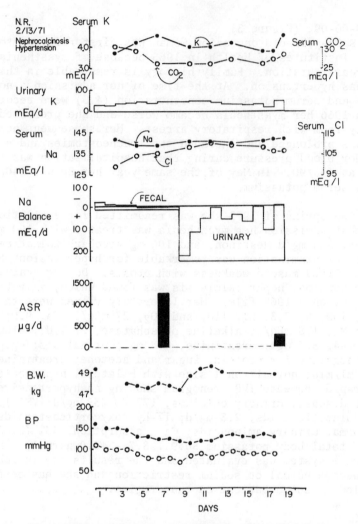

Figure 3.   The effects of low- and high-sodium intakes on serum
            potassium and carbon dioxide concentrations,
            urinary potassium, serum sodium and chloride concent-
            rations, sodium balance, aldosterone secretion rate,
            body weight and blood pressure in a patient, N.R.,
            with nephrocalcinosis.

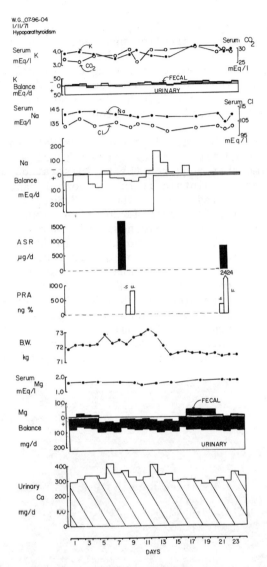

Figure 4.   The effects of high- and low-sodium intakes on serum
potassium and carbon dioxide concentrations, potassium
balance, serum sodium and chloride concentrations,
sodium balance, aldosterone secretion rate, plasma
renin activity, body weight, serum magnesium concentration, magnesium balance and urinary calcium in
patient W.G. with hypoparathyroidism.

His family history is positive in that his mother has nephrolithiasis and his sister has a goiter. In 1968 his physical examination was normal with a BP of 130/70. The pertinent laboratory studies included the following: Na, 140; K, 3.3; Cl, 101; and CO_2, 26 mEq/L; Ca, 7.9 and PO_4, 2.9 mg%; alkaline phosphatase, 54 I.U.; albumin, 4.0 g%; creatinine clearance, 108 ml/min; nephrocalcinosis with a normal IVP; urinary calcium, over 250 mg/d. Diuril was started as therapy for his hypercalciuria and vitamin D and calcium supplements were continued. In February 1970 he developed vitamin D intoxication and all his medications were stopped.

Two months later he was admitted to the National Institutes of Health for the second time. A low serum potassium concentration was noted at this time that required the administration of supplemental potassium in order to maintain it in the normal range. Other pertinent information revealed: serum albumin, 3.8g%; urinalysis: pH, 5.5; sp.gr. 1.021, negative for protein, sugar and acetone; creatinine clearance, 117 ml/min; nephrocalcinosis with normal renal size and calcium absorption, 55% (31-59%, normal). In January, 1971 he was readmitted for further investigation of his renin-aldosterone system. In spite of the change in sodium intake he stayed in potassium and magnesium balance (see Figure 4). His blood pressure remained normal during the entire study and his hypercalciuria was unchanged. As shown in Table III he had an abnormal response to both angiotensin and norepinephrine infusion. A renal biopsy was performed and shows prominent juxtaglomerular apparatus in addition to nephrocalcinosis, interstitial fibrosis and chronic pyelitis (Figure 5).

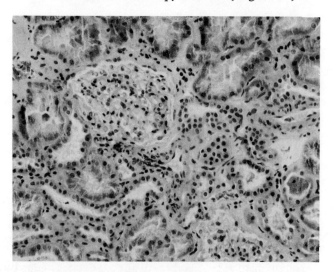

Figure 5. Photomicrograph of a glomerulus in association with its macula densa. Note the hyperplasia of the juxtaglomerular apparatus in patient W.G.

J.M.   02-58-97   (Figure 6)

This 48-year-old caucasian woman was first referred to the Clinical Center in 1958 with the diagnosis of hypoparathyroidism secondary to a thyroid resection in 1944 for a non-toxic nodule. She has required vitamin D and calcium supplementation in addition to thyroid replacement since that time. Her serum calcium has been out of control from time to time and on at least two occasions she developed hypercalcemia with renal impairment. Her family history is positive for diabetes in two siblings.

In 1966 she was admitted to Georgetown University Hospital for recurrent abdominal pain. In addition to a normal gastrointestinal series and barium enema the following findings were recorded: normal physical examination; BP, 126/82; Na, 145; K, 4.2; Cl, 106; CO_2, 22 mEq/L; Ca, 7.8 and PO_4, 4.9 mg%; Mg, 0.2 mEq/L and a diabetic glucose tolerance test. Her low serum magnesium was not fully understood and she was treated with supplemental magnesium for a short time; the hypomagnesemia has not recurred.

In 1967 she was admitted with vitamin D intoxication and reversible renal impairment. In 1968 she was admitted for evaluation of her vitamin D metabolism. In addition to having vitamin D resistance the following observations were made: BP 130/70; Na, 139; K, 3.4; Cl, 106; CO_2, 24 mEq/L; Ca, 8.6 and PO_4, 3.4 mg%; Mg, 1.55 mEq/L; alkaline phosphatase, 46 I.U.; albumin, 3.3 g%; creatinine, 1.5 mg%; BUN, 21 mg%; urinalysis: pH 5.0, negative for protein, sugar and acetone.

In the summer of 1970 she was admitted for a hysterectomy which was complicated with a post-operative infection. Her pertinent data at that time included the following: BP 110/75; Na, 140; K, 3.2; Cl, 102; CO_2, 29 mEq/L; Ca 8.0 and PO_4, 4.1 mg%; alkaline phosphatase, 44 I.U.; albumin, 3.6 g%; BUN, 12 mg%. Because of the frequent previous observations of hypokalemia she was readmitted in the spring of 1971 to evaluate her renin-aldosterone system. During the metabolic balance study she was in slightly negative potassium and magnesium balance; however, her serum potassium concentrations were within the normal range on most occasions. The other pertinent findings are the following: BP 110/70; Ca, 9.0 to 10.0 mg%; PO_4, 4.0 to 4.5 mg%; creatinine 1.2 mg%; urinalysis: pH 5.5, negative for protein, sugar and acetone; creatinine clearance, 70 to 90 ml/min; normal renogram and renal scan; normal rapid sequence IVP; total body potassium, 50.8 mEq/kg (28.7 to 46.0); urinary calcium, 200-400 mg/d. Her responsiveness to angiotensin II and norepinephrine are shown in Table III.

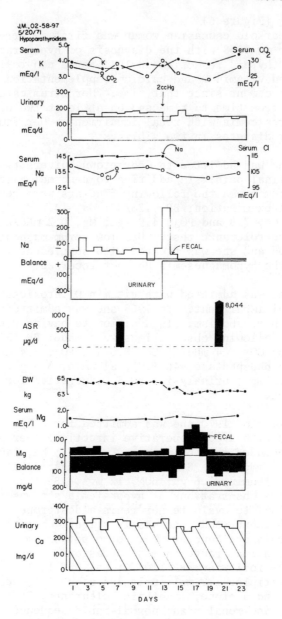

Figure 6.   The effects of high- and low-sodium intakes on the
            serum potassium and carbon dioxide concentrations,
            urinary potassium, serum sodium and chloride concent-
            rations, sodium balance, aldosterone secretion rate,
            body weight, serum magnesium, magnesium balance and
            urinary calcium in patient J.M. with hypopara-
            thyroidism.

RESULTS

Fifty-five patients with hypercalciuria have been seen at this clinic over the past year. The incidence of hypokalemia in this group of patients with hypercalciuria is 12.7 per cent.

The six patients reported are divided into two groups on the basis of their blood pressure. Table II contains the serum K concentration, ASR and PRA on the high sodium intake and the PRA on the low sodium intake in all six patients.

Group I: The four patients in Group I with above-normal PRAs presented with hypokalemia and hypertension and had high aldosterone secretion rates on a high-sodium intake. The investigation of the etiology of the hypertension included the following: normal and equal excretion times in a rapid sequence IVP, normal renograms and normal catecholamines, VMA and 17-hydroxycorticosteroid excretion. Their creatinine clearances range from 90 to 120 ml/min.

None of the patients had a contracted blood volume and none had a "sodium leak" as evidenced by the ability to reduce the urinary sodium below 10 mEq/d. None was potassium-depleted as evidenced by the rapid return of the serum potassium concentrations to normal on low sodium intakes and the normal total body potassium. The patient with the lowest serum potassium concentration in response to the sodium load had a complete metabolic study which shows that this patient is not in negative potassium balance during the twenty four days of her study (Pt. D.B. Figure 2). Two patients (D.B. and N.R., Figure 3) with unexplained nephrocalcinosis became normotensive on a low sodium intake, but neither patient (T.W., Figure 1, or E.B.) who had parathyroidectomy for hyperparathyroidism showed a significant change in his blood pressure with sodium restriction. (Only patient D.B. had recently taken medication which might interfere with the evaluation: 30 days before being studied she had stopped taking Enovid.) All patients demonstrated hyperaldosteronism secondary to increased renins.

Group II: W.G. (Figure 4) and J.M. (Figure 6) have extremely high PRA with normal blood pressure and high ASR on high sodium intakes. Both have had post-operative hypoparathyroidism with resulting hypercalciuria for over 10 years. W.G. had been operated on for hyperparathyroidism and J.M. for removal of a thyroid nodule. Their management has been complicated with episodes of hypercalcemia due to vitamin D intoxication. Both patients have only mild hypokalemia, normal serum magnesium concentrations and completely normal blood pressure. The hypokalemia was corrected by a low sodium intake. Since the diagnosis of Bartter's syndrome was entertained, both patients received infusions of graded doses of angiotensin and norepinephrine to determine the response of blood pressure (Table III) (4). W.G. had an abnormal pressor response to both angiotensin

TABLE II

	Serum K		ASR	Renin		Serum Mg
	Initial	Lowest on 249 Na (mEq/L)	249 Na (μg/day)	S/U 249 Na (ng%)	S/U 9 Na	(mEq/L)
Group I: Hypertensive						
E.B.	3.4	3.4	776	123/635	358/1377	normal
T.W.	3.4	3.7	121	187/345	533/522	normal
D.B.	3.4	3.2	166	331/497	568/ -	normal
N.R.	3.3	3.4	277	*290/ -	579/325	normal
Group II: Normotensive						
W.G.	3.3	3.5	1664	323/780	319/2424	normal
J.M.	3.3	3.5	795	*56/346	2328/3225	normal
Normal		above 3.5	62±28	97±71(S) 212±61(U)	766±478(S) 1369±809(U)	

* Initial sodium intake   30-140/70-250
  "normal", ad libitum.

TABLE III

	Angiotensin* ng/kg/min	Norepinephrine* ng/kg/min
Normal	5 - 10	50 - 100
W.G.	20.8	332
J.M.	11.3	180

* Amount necessary to raise diastolic B.P. 20 mmHg.

and norepinephrine (Table III). J.M.'s response was slightly below
the normal range. Kidney biopsy in W.G. revealed nephrocalcinosis,
interstitual fibrosis, chronic pyelitis and JG hyperplasia
(Figure 5). J.M. did not have a kidney biopsy. W.G. had normal
creatinine clearances and showed nephrocalcinosis on x-ray; J.M.
had slightly reduced creatinine clearances. These patients,
although lacking both profound hypokalemia and hypomagnesemia, seem
to represent a clinical syndrome similar to, but not as severe as
Bartter's syndrome.

DISCUSSION

The association of hypercalciuria and hypokalemia has been
noted in a few isolated case reports of hypercalcemia secondary to
either hyperparathyroidism (5,6) or vitamin D intoxication (7,8).
In these reports the hypokalemia was attributed to kidney damage
resulting from hypercalcemia with resultant potassium wasting.
In many cases the hypokalemia was corrected when the hypercalcemia
was reversed.

The current studies do not support this proposition that the
hypokalemia is associated with kidney damage. In all the patients
reported here there is an abnormality of the renin-aldosterone
system. The patients differ in the blood pressure response: the
first group are hypertensive and the second group are normotensive.

The second group represents the unusual set of circumstances of
normal pressure with increased aldosterone and renin values. This

combination of events has been recorded in four clinical entities:
Bartter's syndrome (9), gastrointestinal potassium loss, potassium
loss resulting from abuse of laxatives (10) or diuretics (11), and
a renal or adrenal tumor (12). In the last-mentioned case report
the patient had an abnormal IVP and abnormal aortogram. The renal
studies in the patients reported here were normal. While on the
metabolic studies, W.G. showed no excess of fecal potassium and a
normal balance, but J.M. lost potassium on a high-sodium intake and
came into balance on the low-sodium intake. The serum potassium
rose into the normal range while the patients were on a low-sodium
diet.

Bartter's syndrome is characterized by massive juxtaglomerular
hyperplasia, normal blood pressure with elevated ASR's and PRA's,
low serum potassium and magnesium concentrations and an abnormal
pressor response to angiotensin. The patients studied here in
group II had mild JG hyperplasia, normal blood pressure, abnormal
pressor responses, mild hypokalemia and normal serum magnesium
concentrations. They had no childhood history of growth retardation,
paralysis, or early episodes of hypokalemia as seen in Bartter's
syndrome. They may represent a mild form of Bartter's syndrome,
an adult or acquired form or perhaps are completely unrelated.

Both groups are examples of hyperaldosteronism secondary to
increased renin activity. The known factors that stimulate renin
secretion include vascular volume depletion (13), potassium depletion (14,15,16), renovascular abnormalities, and certain adrenal
abnormalities such as those seen in the adrenogenital syndrome (17).
The patients clinically did not have a depleted vascular volume:
they all had normal serum albumins, a weight gain with salt loading
and appropriate urinary sodium for the low-sodium diet. The
patients were mildly hypokalemic (serum K concentration from 3.4 to
3.8 mEq/l) when aldosterone secretion rates were determined on the
high-sodium diet: hypokalemia would tend to further lower the ASR's.
Renal vascular abnormalities were ruled out with a rapid-sequence
IVP in all patients and a renogram in some. Adrenal function in all
patients was normal except for the ASR's. The findings do not
provide an explanation for the increased PRA in these patients with
hypercalciuria. It is possible that the increase in calcium in the
distal tubule stimulates the JG apparatus or that the deposited
calcium in the kidney has interfered with the vascular supply to
stimulate directly the JG apparatus or that hypercalciuria and
increased PRA are not directly related. The evidence does not
support any of these hypotheses.

CONCLUSIONS

Patients with hypercalciuria are more likely than the general population to have hypokalemia and an abnormality of the renin-aldosterone system. These patients fall into two groups: increased PRA with secondary aldosteronism and hypertension, and increased. PRA with secondary aldosteronism and normal blood pressure. If there is a role for calcium in stimulating the renin-aldosterone system, it is not explained by the known mechanisms of renin control.

REFERENCES

1. Boucher, R., Veyrat, R., deChamplain, J. and Genest, J.: New procedures for measurement of human plasma angiotensin and renin activity levels. Canad. Med. Assoc. J. 90:194, 1964.

2. Haber, E., Koerner, T., Page, L.B., Kliman, B. and Purnode, A.: Application of a radioimmunoassay for angiotensin I to the physiologic measurements of plasma renin activity in normal human subjects. J. Clin. Endocr. 29:1349, 1969.

3. Wills, M.R., Zisman, E., Wortsman, J., Evens, R.G., Pak, C.Y.C. and Bartter, F.C.: The measurement of intestinal calcium absorption by external radioisotope counting: application to study of nephrolithiasis. Clin. Sci. 39:95, 1970.

4. Gill, J.R., Jr., and Bartter, F.C.: Hyperplasia of the juxtaglomerular complex with hyperaldosteronism and hypokalemic alkalosis. In: Water and Electrolyte Metabolism (II), J. de Graeff and B. Leijnse (Editors) Elsevier Publishing Co., Amsterdam, 1964, p. 119.

5. Bottiger, L.E.: Hypopotassemia in hyperparathyroidism. Acta Med. Scand. 148:51, 1954.

6. Sanderson, P.H.: Renal potassium wasting in hypercalcaemia. Brit. Med. J. 1:679, 1967.

7. Anderson, D.C., Cooper, A.F. and Naylor, G.J.: Vitamin D intoxication with hypernatremia, potassium and water depletion, and mental depression. Brit. Med. J. 4:744, 1968.

8. Ferris, T.F., Levitin, H., Phillips, E.T. and Epstein, F.H.: Renal potassium-wasting induced by vitamin D. J. Clin. Invest. 41:1222, 1962.

9. Bartter, F.C., Pronove, P., Gill, J.R., Jr., and MacCardle, R.C.: Hyperplasia of the juxtaglomerular complex with hyperaldosteronism and hypokalemic alkalosis. A new syndrome. Am. J. Med. 33: 811, 1962.

10. Fleisher, N., Brown, H., Graham, D., Delena, S.: Chronic laxative induced hyperaldosteronism and hypokalemia simulating Bartter's syndrome. Ann. Int. Med. 70:791, 1969.

11. Wolff, H.P., Kruck, F., Brown, J.J., Lever, A.F., Vecsei, P., Roscher, S., Dusterdieck, G.O., and Robertson, J.I.S.: Psychiatric disturbance leading to potassium depletion, sodium depletion, raised plasma-renin concentration and secondary hyperaldosteronism. The Lancet 1:257, 1968.

12. Fichman, M.P., Crane, M.G. and Bethune, J.E.: Hypokalemia with normal blood pressure, aldosterone and renin levels secondary to a renal or adrenal tumor. Amer. J. Med. 48:509, 1970.

13. Newsome, H.H. and Bartter, F.C.: Plasma renin activity in relation to sodium concentration and body fluid balance. J. Clin. Endocr. 28:1704, 1968.

14. Abbrecht, P.H. and Vander, A.J.: Effects of chronic potassium deficiency on plasma renin activity. J. Clin. Invest. 49:1510, 1970.

15. Sealey, J.E., Clark, I., Bull, M.B. and Laragh, J.H.: Potassium balance and the control of renin secretion. J. Clin. Invest. 49:2119, 1970.

16. Brunner, H.R., Baer, L., Sealey. J.E., Ledingham, J.G.G. and Laragh, J.H.: The influence of potassium administration and of potassium deprivation on plasma renin in normal and hypertensive subjects. J. Clin. Invest. 49:2128, 1970.

17. Simopoulos, A.P., Marshall, J.R., Delea, C.S. and Bartter, F.C.: Studies on the deficiency of 21-hydroxylation in patients with congenital adrenal hyperplasia. J. Clin. Endocr. Metab. 32:438, 1971.

ADDENDUM

Since the preparation of the manuscript, Dr. Andrew M. Michelakis in "The Effect of Sodium and Calcium on Renin Release in Vitro.", Proc. Soc. Exptl. Biol. Med. 137:833, 1971, demonstrated that renin release is enhanced from renal slices by increasing the calcium concentration in the medium. These data and the above paper indicate that the role of calcium in the release of renin should be investigated further.

ACUTE CIRCULATORY RENAL FAILURE: A PROBABLE MANIFESTATION OF EXCESS RENIN RELEASE

J.J. Brown, H. Gavras, B. Leckie, A.F. Lever,

R. MacAdam, J.J. Morton, and J.I.S. Robertson

Medical Research Council, Blood Pressure Unit, Western

Infirmary, Glasgow, W.1., Scotland

The earliest studies of renin (Tigerstedt & Bergman, 1898) were largely concerned with its possible role as a hormone, released from the kidney into blood, and acting on distant target organs. Hitherto, the greater bulk of work on renin, and on its active product, the peptide angiotensin, has been concentrated on this hormonal function, principally on the pressor (Tigerstedt & Bergman, 1898; Pickering & Prinzmetal, 1938; Brown et al., 1967), and aldosterone-stimulating effects (Gross, 1958, 1960; Genest et al., 1960; Laragh et al., 1960; Davis, 1961; Mulrow & Ganong, 1961), and to a lesser extent on the thirst-provoking (Fitzsimons & Simons, 1969) and other actions.

The effects of renin and angiotensin on renal function, although well-recognised (Pickering & Prinzmetal 1940; De Bono et al., 1963; Bock et al., 1968) have attracted rather less atten-tion, partly because of the difficulty in examining these in isola-tion. However, as we have considered previously (Brown et al., 1968), the renin-angiotensin system might well phylogenetically have been concerned primarily with intrarenal functions, and the peripheral actions could have been acquired later in the course of evolution. (The somewhat different, but by no means conflicting view, that the aldosterone-stimulating role of renin is deeply-rooted phylogenetically, is considered at length by Davis (1971) in a recent review).

In the present paper, we shall be concerned with the direct renal actions of renin and angiotensin, and, in particular, shall consider the evidence that stimuli activating such renal actions

may, if sufficiently intense and prolonged, lead to excessive
release of renin, to disadvantageous renal effects and, in extreme
instances, to acute circulatory renal failure. We shall consider
also evidence on whether such renal effects are due to angiotensin
formed within the kidney, or whether release of renin into the
systemic circulation is required, the effective concentration of
the octapeptide angiotensin II then reaching the kidney in arterial
blood.

Acute, potentially reversible, impairment of renal function
is, in man, usually associated with oliguria, and several author-
ities (e.g. De Wardener, 1963) define acute renal failure in terms
of reduction in urine flow rate below a certain arbitrary figure.
In experimental animals, however (see Finckh et al., 1962),
oliguria is a less common feature, and the severity and progress of
the disease can more reliably be assessed by the impairment of
excretion of urea or creatinine, as may be reflected in a fall in
urine/plasma urea and creatinine ratios. It is now also clear that
acute renal failure is not necessarily associated with renal histological abnormalities, at least as judged by light microscopy;
moreover, histologically evident acute tubular necrosis is not
always accompanied by acute renal failure (Brun & Munck, 1957;
Sevitt, 1959; Finckh et al., 1962; Brown et al., 1970a; Gavras et
al., 1971a).

When clear histological abnormalities are found in acute
renal failure, it is possible to define two broad aetiological
groups (Oliver et al., 1951; De Wardener, 1963):- "circulatory"
or "ischaemic" as following haemorrhage, hypotension, renal artery
obstruction, haemolysis, etc; and "nephrotoxic", as produced by the
administration of salts of mercury and uranium, certain antibiotics
etc. Renal tubular lesions are often widespread in the "circulatory" variety, and may involve proximal, distal, and collecting
tubules. The tubular basement membrane may be disrupted, exposing
interstitial tissue to the tubular lumen. Visible glomerular
lesions are unusual, although Clarkson et al. (1970), on the basis
of electron microscopic studies, obtained evidence of intraglomer-
ular capillary thrombosis, and considered the possible contribution
of this to the functional renal impairment. In the "nephrotoxic"
variety, by contrast, the lesions are usually localised to the
proximal tubules, and the basement membrane is rarely, if ever,
affected.

The nature of the major intrarenal event leading to the
impairment of renal function has been the subject of much investigation and speculation; reduction in renal blood flow and glomerular filtration, and obstruction, necrosis and increased permeabil-
ity of renal tubules have all been considered. To date, however,
there is no general agreement on the primary feature. Nevertheless, despite the difficulty of accurate measurement in this

disease, which precludes the use of clearance techniques, there is
no doubt of a marked reduction in renal blood flow (to about 1/3
normal; see Ladefoged & Munck, 1971) and in glomerular filtration
rate.

The possibility that the oliguria in such diseases as the
crush syndrome and eclampsia might result from constriction of
glomerular vessels caused by renin liberated from the juxtaglomerular cells of the afferent arteriole was considered by Goormaghtigh
(1942, 1945, 1947) on the basis of the increased granularity of
these cells which he observed. The present paper will be concerned
with more recent clinical and experimental evidence on the aetiological relationship of renin to acute renal failure, and the
therapeutic implications of the findings. As will be seen, both
factual and circumstantial evidence links renin more closely with
circulatory forms of acute renal failure, although it should be
emphasised that a major or contributory role of renin to the
nephrotoxic form is not excluded on present evidence.

Clinical Acute Renal Failure:
Circumstantial Evidence Implicating Renin and Angiotensin

Goormaghtigh (1942, 1945, 1947) noted increased granularity
of the cells of the afferent glomerular arterioles in patients with
the crush syndrome and eclampsia. These granules are now confirmed
as the normal storage site of renin (Cook, 1971). Goormaghtigh
proposed that this increased cellular granularity probably indicated increased activity of the renin-angiotensin system, and that
consequent constriction of glomerular vessels might be responsible
for the oliguria.

A variety of clinical states which cause or predispose to
acute renal failure are now known to be associated with increased
concentrations of renin in plasma and in the kidney. These
include sodium depletion, hypovolaemia, severe cardiac failure,
hepatic cirrhosis with ascites, Addison's disease, pregnancy and
renal allotransplantation (see Brown et al., 1966a, 1970a, 1970b;
also Schroeder et al., 1970; Roguska et al., 1971). Conversely,
sodium loading reduces both the renal renin content (see Gross
et al., 1964) and plasma renin concentration (Brown et al., 1964b)
and protects against experimental acute renal failure (Teschan &
Lawson, 1966; Wilson et al., 1967; Henry et al., 1968). Similarly,
denervation of the kidney reduces its renin content (Ueda et al.,
1967), and has been suggested as protecting the kidney against
acute failure (Powers et al., 1957).

More direct evidence has been obtained from measurement of
circulating renin and angiotensin in acute ischaemic renal failure.

Increases in serum or plasma renin activity have been reported by
Tu (1965), Kokot & Kuska (1969) and Roguska et al. (1971); in
plasma renin concentration by Schröder et al. (1969) and Brown et
al. (1970a); and in whole blood angiotensin level by Massani et al.
(1966) and Ochoa et al. (1970). Serial renin measurements in
individual cases were reported in the papers of Kokot & Kuska
(1969) and Brown et al. (1970a) and demonstrated that while
abnormally high plasma levels occurred during the oliguric phase,
these declined towards or into the normal range with recovery of
renal function. Figure 1 shows the data of Brown et al. (1970a).

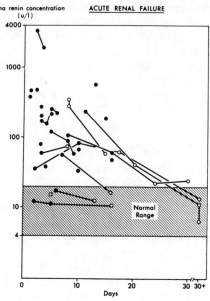

Figure 1.   47 estimations of plasma renin concentration in 25
            patients with acute renal failure. Log. ordinate
            scale. Abscissa shows duration of disease. Empty
            circles indicate values at a time when daily urine
            volume was greater than 1 litre; solid circles values
            when urine volume was less than this. Lines join
            serial estimates from same patient.

In only three of twenty-five patients were abnormally high plasma
renin levels not found at some stage. Two of these were in acute
renal failure associated with pregnancy and it is noteworthy that
measurement of plasma renin concentration alone may be an inadequate index of stimulation of the renin-angiotensin system in
pregnancy, owing to the considerable increase in renin-substrate
level in that condition (Helmer & Judson, 1967; Robertson et al.,
1971). The third example was of diconal poisoning. It is perhaps
also worthy of comment that all three patients with normal renin
levels survived the acute renal failure.

The development of radioimmunoassay methods for the measurement of plasma angiotensin II concentration has permitted more
specific study than was possible in the paper by Massani et al.
(1966), which did not distinguish between angiotensin I and II.
Figure 2 shows angiotensin II levels, measured by the technique of
Düsterdieck and McElwee (1971) in a patient who developed acute
renal failure after the insertion of a Dacron aortic bifurcation
graft. The operation was followed by the development of a lung
abscess which was treated with cephaloridine. As can be seen, the
initial plasma angiotensin II concentration in this man was roughly
four times the normal upper limit, subsequent values falling within
the normal range. The case also exemplifies the multiple aetiological factors often concerned in clinical acute renal failure,
making interpretation of the pathogenic role of angiotensin
difficult.

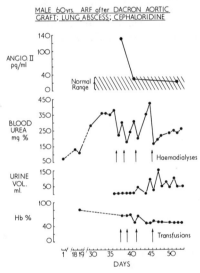

Figure 2.   Peripheral plasma angiotensin II measurements in a
            patient with acute renal failure following the inser-
            tion of a Dacron aortic bifurcation graft, and with
            post-operative lung abscess, treated with cephaloridine.

The evidence summarised so far shows that renin and angiotensin are consistently elevated in acute renal failure, and thus
provides a possible explanation of the reduced renal blood flow
and glomerular filtration rate. It is however, inconclusive,
since several interpretations are possible. Firstly, the elevation
in circulating renin and angiotensin might be a consequence rather
than a cause of the renal failure, either from excessive renin
secretion or diminished renal clearance, or a combination of the
two. Secondly, increased renin secretion and acute renal failure

might be provoked independently of each other by some as yet
undefined stimulus. These require to be considered before the
third contingency, that the increase in renin is the cause of the
acute renal failure, can be more firmly established. Further
studies along these lines were therefore conducted using experimental animal models.

Glycerol-Induced Renal Failure in the Rabbit

In this study the experimental model extensively used by Oken
and his colleagues for the production of acute circulatory renal
failure in the rat (see Oken et al., 1966) was employed in the
rabbit. Renal failure and tubular necrosis were induced by a
subcutaneous injection by glycerol, arterial plasma renin concentration being measured before and 6, 24 or 72 hours from the injection (Brown et al., 1970a, 1971b). The quantity of renin extractable from whole kidneys and from individual glomeruli was also
measured.

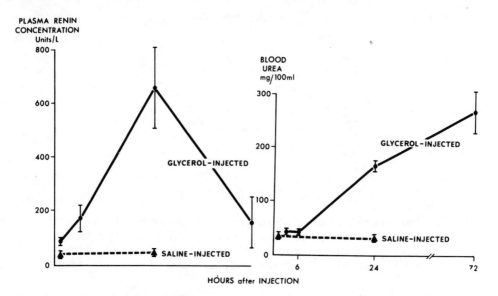

Figure 3.   Changes in plasma renin concentration and blood urea 6,
             24 and 72 hours after glycerol injection in rabbits
             (means ± SEM). Values in saline-injected controls
             shown for comparison.

Figure 3 summarises the results of the plasma renin and urea
estimation. There was no significant increase in mean blood urea
6 hours after glycerol injection, but a marked and progressive
elevation was found in the mean levels at 24 and 72 hours. As can

be seen from Figure 3, the increase and peak level of plasma renin
concentration slightly preceded this course of change in urea. A
distinct rise in mean plasma renin was already apparent 6 hours
after glycerol administration, with a maximum at 24 hours. The
mean 72 hour renin level had fallen to roughly the 6 hour value,
although mean blood urea was still increasing at this time. No
changes in renin or urea were seen in saline-injected control
rabbits.

   The results of renal renin estimation in this series of
animals are of considerable interest in relation to Goormaghtigh's
(1945, 1947) observation of increased cellularity of the juxtaglomerular apparatus in acute renal failure. Both the total
extractable renin and the quantity associated with individual
glomeruli were significantly lower in the glycerol-injected rabbits
with acute renal failure than in the controls. The reduction in
glomerular renin was more striking in the superficial zone of the
renal cortex, where the glomerular renin content is normally much
higher than in the deep cortex (Brown et al., 1965). This reduction of renal and glomerular renin further suggested that the
increase in peripheral plasma renin concentration in acute renal
failure was a consequence of discharge of renin from the kidney
into the blood. While a reduction of renin synthesis could account
for the depletion of kidney renin, it could not explain the
increased renin content of blood.

   These experiments therefore produced results which appeared
compatible with the notion that renin is involved in the pathogenesis of acute renal failure. The relative timing of the
increases in circulating renin and urea seemed particularly suggestive, and the absence of significant changes in the control
animals excluded haemorrhage as a cause of either the renal failure
or the increase in renin. Not eliminated however, was the possibility that renin and renal failure were stimulated independently
by a common factor such as haemolysis. That the increase in plasma
renin was a consequence of renal impairment, although unlikely from
a consideration of the relative timing of the peak levels of renin
and urea, was also still possible. In an attempt to clarify some
of these points a further series of studies was performed with a
rather different experimental design.

Cephaloridine-Induced Renal Failure in the Rabbit

   Cephaloridine is a polypeptide antibiotic with marked nephro-
toxicity in the rabbit. In this series of experiments acute renal
failure and proximal tubular necrosis were induced in rabbits by
means of a single large intramuscular injection of cephaloridine
(500 mg/Kg), a control series of animals being given intramuscular

dextrose. Serial blood samples were obtained from all animals 24
hours before and 2, 24 and 72 hours after injection (Gavras et al.,
1971b).

    All rabbits receiving cephaloridine developed severe renal
failure, with extensive necrosis localised to proximal convoluted
tubules. The rise in blood urea was very similar in course and
severity to that in glycerol-induced renal failure. The changes in
plasma renin were, however, very different (Figure 4).

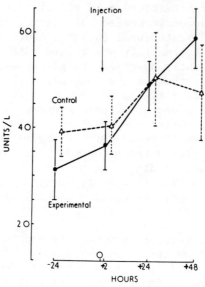

Figure 4.   Plasma renin concentration before and after injection
            of cephaloridine (circles) and in control rabbits
            injected with dextrose (triangles). (means ± SEM).

Only minor and inconsistent increases in renin were found, and
there was no significant difference in renin levels between the
experimental and control groups. In 6 of the 16 rabbits develop-
ing acute renal failure, there was no detectable increase in
plasma renin concentration at any stage. The slight increase seen
in mean plasma renin concentration in both groups was thought possibly to be attributable to the relatively large blood samples
taken and to negative sodium balance which developed in the
cephaloridine-injected animals.

    These experiments established that severe nephrotoxic renal
failure could develop in the absence of an increase in peripheral
plasma renin concentration, and moreover, provided no evidence
that renin might be involved in this form of the disease. It was

also established that acute renal failure does not necessarily lead
to an increase in plasma renin concentration. However, renin was
not excluded as a pathogenic factor, since it could well be that
cephaloridine caused a marked reduction in renal blood flow, which
might have resulted in a rise in intrarenal renin in the absence of
appreciable changes in the peripheral circulation. More direct
evidence on this point was provided by measurement of renal venous
renin in rabbits in which acute tubular necrosis was provoked by
renal artery clamping.

Acute Tubular Necrosis Induced by Renal Artery Occlusion in Rabbits

In these animals the left renal vein and central ear artery
were cannulated under general anaesthesia, and the left renal
artery occluded by clamping for 4 hours. Samples of arterial and
renal venous blood were obtained before and at the end of the
period of renal artery occlusion and again 24 hours later, after
which the animals were killed and the kidneys examined histologically (Brown et al., 1971b).

Renal artery clamping for 4 hours consistently produced
extensive necrosis involving proximal, distal and collecting
tubules, with the addition of cortical infarction in 8 rabbits.
The opposite untouched kidneys were free from these abnormalities.

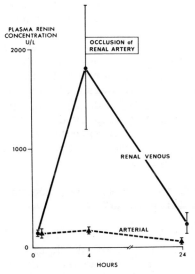

Figure 5. Changes of arterial and renal venous plasma renin
concentration produced by a 4-hour period of renal
artery occlusion in 11 rabbits (means ± SEM).

The changes in renal venous and arterial plasma renin concentration are summarised in Figure 5. Renal venous plasma renin concentration increased in all animals during renal artery occlusion, from 1.14- to 34-fold, with a mean increase of 12-fold. Lower values were found 20 hours after the clamp had been released. Mean arterial plasma renin concentration, by contrast, did not increase significantly during the occlusion. Thus, in the presence of severe reduction of renal blood flow, a very marked increase in intrarenal renin level may occur in the absence of a detectable change in the arterial level.

Renal Failure and Tubular Necrosis Induced by Angiotensin Infusion

Notwithstanding the body of evidence favouring a pathogenic role for renin and angiotensin in acute "circulatory" or "ischaemic" renal failure, a considerable obstacle to the hypothesis was doubt concerning the ability of administered angiotensin to produce the disease.

Byrom (1964) made extensive studies in both anaesthetised and unanaesthetised rats, administering angiotensin II intravenously as 1-100 μg injections and 0.01-5.0 μg per minute infusions, without producing renal tubular necrosis. These results contrasted with the evidence that several other vasoconstrictor substances, such as adrenaline, serotonin, pitressin and oxytocin, and even, possibly, crude renal extracts, can cause renal failure and tubular or cortical necrosis (see Brown et al, 1970a).

However, Brown et al (1964a) found that while angiotensin II could be infused intravenously to conscious rabbits in a dose range of 0.057 to 0.136 μg per Kg per minute for up to 100 days without causing uraemia, three animals given larger doses (0.350-0.455 μg per Kg per minute for 3-10 days) developed a striking increase in blood urea, together with evidence of tubular necrosis. Because of these findings the renal effects of large intravenous infusions of angiotensin in the rabbit were examined in more detail (Gavras et al, 1971a).

Three groups of rabbits were studied, sodium and potassium balances being computed daily in all.

In the first group of 5, a control infusion of 0.9% saline was given for 72 hours, at the end of which time peripheral arterial blood was taken for urea and electrolyte estimation. Angiotensin II (0.9-1.8 μg per Kg per minute) was then infused for a further 72 hours, additional blood samples being drawn daily for

urea and electrolyte measurement. The animals were then killed
and the kidneys and heart examined histologically. Angiotensin
caused a steep rise in blood urea, which was apparent within 24
hours, and reached levels around 200 mg per 100 ml at 48 hours
(Figure 6). Accompanying this was a distinct fall in the urine/
plasma ratios of both urea and creatinine. Angiotensin infusion
also caused a negative balance of both sodium and potassium. Post-
mortem, the kidneys of 3 of these 5 rabbits showed widespread
tubular necrosis of the "ischaemic" or "circulatory" type, involving proximal, distal and collecting tubules.

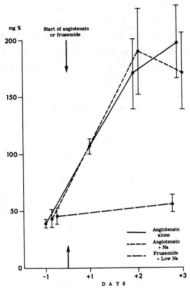

Figure 6.   Blood urea levels (means ± SEM) before and at daily
             intervals after starting intravenous infusion of angio-
             tensin II at high dose. Solid line indicates angioten-
             sin infusion alone; dotted line angiotensin infusion
             with saline supplements. Also shown (dashed line) are
             blood urea values in rabbits sodium depleted for 3 days,
             but not infused with angiotensin.

    Because of the natriuresis induced by these large doses of
angiotensin II, it was necessary to exclude the possibility of the
changes in renal structure and function being the result of sodium
deficiency. A further series of 5 rabbits was therefore studied
in the same way, except that a subcutaneous injection of saline
was given immediately before the start of the angiotensin infusion, and repeated daily so as to maintain positive sodium balance
throughout. The changes in renal function were clearly similar to
those observed in the first group (Figure 6) and all 5 developed
renal tubular necrosis.

A third group of 5 rabbits was placed on a sodium-deficient diet and given daily intramuscular injections of 20 mg furosemide so as to produce within 72 hours a cumulative sodium and potassium deficit slightly in excess of that of the first group infused with angiotensin. No impairment of renal function was observed in this third group (Figure 6), and no histological changes were found in their kidneys.

The changes in renal function were therefore unrelated to alterations in sodium balance; nor could they be attributed to haemorrhage; and it is clear that the intravenous administration of large doses of angiotensin II to rabbits can consistently produce both the biochemical and histological features of acute renal failure. The tubular lesions found appeared to be of varying ages, with evidence of resolution in places. Histologically, they closely resembled those in the glycerol-injected rabbits (Brown et al., 1971b), and were quite distinct from those in the cephaloridine-injected animals, where the abnormalities were localised to proximal tubules. No arteriolar lesions could be seen on light microscopy in the kidneys of the angiotensin-infused rabbits, another point of contrast with rats of Byrom's (1964) experiments.

A quite unexpected finding in the rabbits infused with angio-tensin was the presence of widespread focal myocardial infarction, which was seen in 6 of the 7 angiotensin-infused rabbits in which the hearts were examined post-mortem (Figure 7). These myocardial lesions were not present in the furosemide-injected sodium - depleted rabbits nor in a further control group of 5 rabbits bled to a similar extent over 72 hours. However, a more careful exam-ination of the myocardium post-mortem in rabbits with renal fail-ure following glycerol injection has consistently shown widespread focal myocardial infarction closely similar to that following angiotensin infusion.

Angiotensin and Clinical Myocardial Infarction

The frequent occurrence of focal myocardial infarction in rabbits infused with large doses of angiotensin raises the problem of whether high circulating concentrations of angiotensin ever lead to myocardial ischaemia in clinical situations in man. In this connexion, two recent cases studied in our own wards may be of interest.

The first was a 27 year old woman with bilateral progressive pyelonephritis and chronic renal failure. She had presented one year previously with malignant phase hypertension, and the blood pressure remained very difficult to control with hypotensive drugs. Because of worsening uraemia, haemodialysis was performed. Immed-iately before dialysis, peripheral plasma angiotensin II

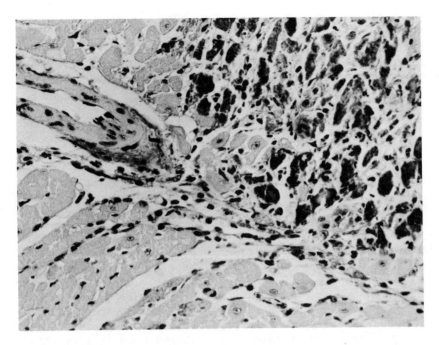

Figure 7.   Photomicrograph showing focal myocardial infarction
            (top right) in rabbit infused with angiotensin.
            (H & E x 350).

concentration was 138 pg/ml (normal range 5 - 35 pg/ml). During
haemodialysis cardiac arrest occurred, and the patient died 24
hours later. Post-mortem, recent widespread microscopic focal
myocardial infarction was found, together with atheroma, but not
thrombosis, in the main coronary arteries. The possibility that
haemodialysis might have stimulated renin release and thereby
increased the already abnormally high plasma angiotensin concentration to a point where myocardial ischaemia occurred, seems worthy
of consideration.

    The second case was a 52 year old female with malignant phase
hypertension and renal impairment (blood urea 152 mg/100 ml).
Plasma angiotensin II levels in peripheral venous blood on admission were 71 and 125 pg/ml. Renal function rapidly deteriorated,
and despite peritoneal dialysis, she died 10 days later. As in
the first patient, widespread recent microscopic focal myocardial
infarction was found post mortem, together with a larger infarct
involving the interventricular septum. The coronary arteries were
free from atheroma.

    Thus both these patients were known to have high circulating
levels of angiotensin II and in both myocardial infarction was

observed, similar in distribution and histology to the lesions in rabbits infused with angiotensin. Although no more than suggestive, these 2 examples seem on present evidence to be consistent with the suggestion that high circulating levels of angiotensin may sometimes have adverse myocardial effects in clinical situations.

Relative Importance of Systemic Arterial Versus Intrarenal Angiotensin II

The evidence summarised in the preceding pages constitutes a strong, but not conclusive case suggesting a pathogenic role for renin and angiotensin II in acute ischaemic renal failure. The relation to the nephrotoxic variety is more tenuous. In order to carry the argument further, more detailed quantitative measurements of angiotensin reaching renal tissues are required. For example, a comparison of peripheral arterial angiotensin II concentrations in acute renal failure induced by subcutaneous glycerol with those in renal failure provoked by angiotensin infusion should indicate whether the concentration of angiogensin II reaching the kidney in arterial blood is likely to be critical. We are at present examining this question. The possibility that angiotensin II might require to reach the kidney by this route in order to affect renal function was raised by the findings of Ng and Vane (1968) in the dog. These workers observed that transit through the pulmonary circulation was necessary for the conversion of the presumably inactive decapeptide angiotensin I to the active octapeptide angiotensin II in any quantity.

However, the wholly intrarenal formation of angiotensin II remains a potentially important possibility in the present context. In earlier studies (Hosie et al., 1970) a significant inverse relationship was demonstrated between renal blood flow and renal venous plasma renin concentration, and we have also shown that severe reduction of renal blood flow by renal artery clamping can lead to a very big increase in renal venous plasma renin level, and to tubular necrosis, in the absence of a significant rise in arterial plasma renin (Brown et al., 1971b); Figure 5).

Several separate lines of evidence suggest that angiotensin II can be formed wholly within the kidney. Thus Oparil et al. (1970) found that a proportion of labelled angiotensin I injected into the renal artery of a dog could be recovered as angiotensin II in the renal vein. In this connexion it should be borne in mind that Akinkugbe et al. (1966) in the rabbit, and Ng and Vane (1968) in the dog, found that angiotensin II was rapidly inactivated in a single passage through the renal circulation.

TABLE I

Patient	Normal renal vein	Artery	Stenotic side renal vein
S.S.	26	29	32
C.M.	20	35	51
M.M.	34	50	54
O.P.	78	210	213
C.N.	9.5	6.5	6.5
C.W.	7.7	4.7	7.7
S.W.	30	34	239

Legend. Plasma angiotensin II (pg/ml) in renal veins and artery in 7 cases of renal artery stenosis. Samples obtained by catheter under local anaesthesia in recumbent subjects. In each case the mean values of several samples are shown. Note that, except in the two patients with low angiotensin levels (C.N. and C.W.), angiotensin II concentration was consistently higher in plasma obtained from the renal vein of the kidney with the stenotic renal artery, and consistently lower in that from the contralateral normal side, than in arterial plasma.

Using radioimmunoassay methods for the measurement of angiotensin II, Sundsfjord (1969) and Gocke et al. (1969) found that in certain situations in man, the concentration of angiotensin II in the renal venous plasma might exceed that in simultaneously-sampled arterial plasma. Our own results in cases of renal artery stenosis (Table I) confirm these observations; also, like Gocke et al. (1969), we have found often lower levels of angiotensin II in renal venous plasma draining the contralateral kidney than in arterial plasma. Interestingly, Bailie et al. (1971) found in the dog that angiotensin II concentration in renal venous plasma always remained below that in arterial plasma, even when the levels were increased following haemorrhage.

Carrière & Biron (1970) were able to demonstrate distinct effects on renal function in the dog on administration of

angiotensin I into one renal artery, although the contralateral
kidney remained unaffected. This clearly implies intrarenal conversion of angiotensin I to II within the kidney, unless angiotensin I has a direct renal action of its own.

Thurau et al. (1970) reported the formation of angiotensin II
on incubation of renin substrate with rat glomeruli. Studies with
a rather different experimental design, performed in our own laboratories by Leckie, Gavras, McGregor and McElwee (unpublished)
have also demonstrated that the incubation of angiotensin I for
48 hours with isolated superficial and deep glomeruli at 37°C and
pH 5.7, results in partial conversion to angiotensin II, and that
this conversion cannot be attributed to contamination of the glomerular tissues with blood (Figure 8). These experiments do not
provide quantitative evidence of the in vivo rate of conversion of
angiotensin I, but they establish the feasibility of intrarenal
formation of angiotensin II.

Finally, the possibility that intrarenal effects of renin and
angiotensin may, at least in part, be mediated by way of renal
lymph, must be considered. Lever and Peart (1962) demonstrated
the presence of high concentrations of renin, together with small
quantities of renin-substrate, in renal lymph of dogs. More
recently, Bailie et al. (1971) have employed radioimmunoassay to
identify angiotensin II in dog renal lymph.

Renal Blood Flow Changes, Acute Renal
Failure, and Angiotensin

Current techniques for the estimation of overall renal blood
flow and intrarenal blood flow changes have recently been reviewed
critically by Ladefoged and Munck (1971). These workers, and also
Barger (1966) and Barger & Herd (1971) have, in addition, considered renal blood flow changes occurring in various clinical and
experimental situations.

There is general agreement that overall renal blood flow is
reduced to about 1/3 normal in acute renal failure. Less severe
impairment of renal blood flow probably occurs in situations pre-
disposing to acute renal failure, such as cardiac failure, hepatic
cirrhosis and haemorrhage. There is also evidence for a selective
cortical ischaemia in acute renal failure, congestive cardiac
failure, renal artery stenosis, renal allotransplants and possibly
hepatic cirrhosis. It is to be emphasized that this does not imply
an increase in medullary flow, only that the reduction affects the
cortex preferentially. While some workers have reported a similar
selective reduction in cortical blood flow during haemorrhage,

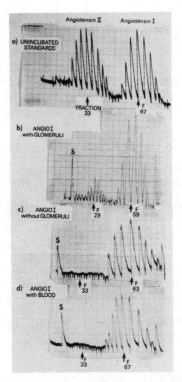

Figure 8.   Conversion of angiotensin I to II by incubation with
            rabbit glomeruli. Blood pressure responses (in mm Hg)
            to intravenous injections in anaesthetised rat. Panel
            (a) shows separation of angiotensins I and II by
            Sephadex chromatography; (b) Formation of angiotensin
            II on incubation of angiotensin I with glomeruli; (c)
            and (d) demonstrate respectively absence of conversion
            in absence of glomeruli; and in presence of quantities
            of rabbit blood contained in glomeruli. "S" indicates
            injection of angiotensin standard.

this is not generally agreed, and the probable consensus of
opinion currently is that the renal blood flow is reduced homogen-
eously in haemorrhagic hypotensin.

    The effects of administered angiotensin on renal blood flow
are also disputed. While there is little doubt of an overall
reduction in flow, the evidence for selective cortical ischaemia
is less uniform. However, the angiographic studies of Daniel et
al. (1954) in which, in the rabbit, injected renin was seen to
produce selective vasoconstriction in the peripheral renal cortex,
are noteworthy. Whatever the merits of the various arguments, it
should be emphasized that the distribution of renin within the

kidney is unequal, the cortical glomeruli being richest in associated renin. Further, the vascular and macula densa structure
differs greatly at different levels within the cortex (see Brown
et al., 1965). Consequently, both the quantity of renin available,
and probably the stimuli leading to its release, could well vary
so as to lead to quite marked selective cortical ischaemia when
endogenous angiotensin formation, as opposed to exogenous administration, is involved.

      We have previously considered in some detail various hypo-
thetical mechanisms whereby pathologically large concentrations of
angiotensin II might be formed in the glomerular region in acute
renal failure (Brown et al., 1970a), and have emphasized that this
could result from increased renin release, or from reduced glomerular blood flow with constant renin release, or, more probably,
from a combination of the two (Figure 9). As we have pointed out,
a critical point would be reached when angiotensin reached sufficient concentration to reduce renal blood flow, since further
increases in angiotensin would then reduce renal blood flow even
more, and a vicious cycle would have been established.

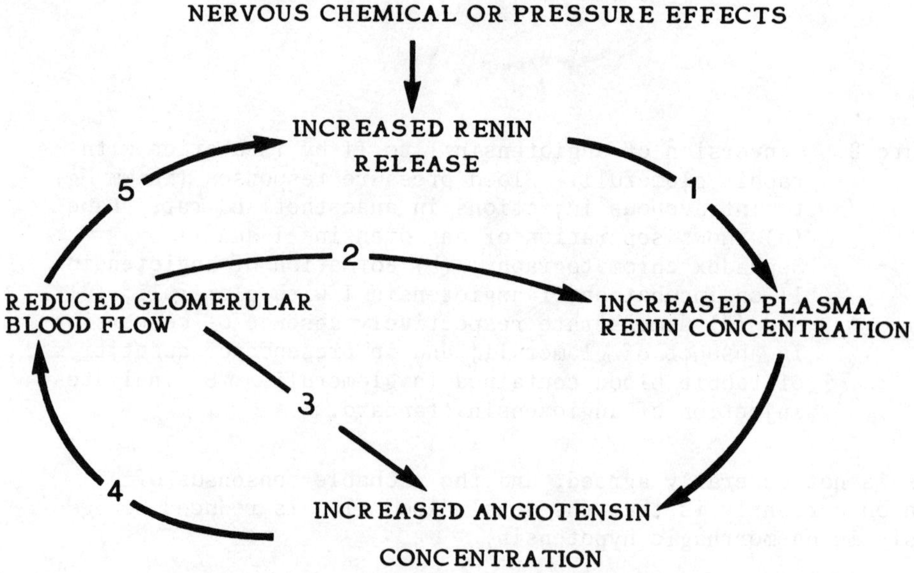

Figure 9.   Schematic representation of 3 ways in which increased
            concentration of angiotensin might be produced in
            glomerular region.

The very high intrarenal concentrations of angiotensin would then,
it is suggested, lead to constriction of afferent glomerular
arterioles and/or glomerular capillaries, with reduction of glomerular filtration and peritubular blood flow, oliguria and, in severe

instances, tubular or cortical necrosis. If these notions have
any validity, clearly measurements of renin and angiotensin in
renal venous plasma are, as we have discussed earlier, more
relevant than those in peripheral blood.

Acute Circulatory Renal Failure as the Pathological
Extreme of a Normal Physiological Response

If we can assume for present purposes that angiotensin II can
be formed within the kidney, and accept as probable that abnormally
high intrarenal levels of angiotensin II are responsible at least
in part for the reduction in renal blood flow and glomerular filtration of "circulatory" renal failure, it is possible to speculate
on the reasons why this situation arises. It seems likely, as we
have discussed elsewhere, (Brown et al., 1970a) that acute circulatory or ischaemic renal failure is the pathological extreme of a
normal physiological response to an embarrassed renal circulation.
Assuming that release of renin from juxtaglomerular cells normally
parallels the graded distribution within the renal cortex, and
that some intrarenal formation of angiotensin II occurs in blood,
then the intrarenal vessels downstream from the juxtamedullary
deep glomeruli, such as the vasa recta loops, are normally subject
to little or no vasoconstrictor effect of angiotensin. By contrast,
the smaller superficial glomeruli, presumably from their anatomical
position more distal in the arterial tree, being perfused at somewhat lower afferent arteriolar pressure than the deep glomeruli,
would release rather greater concentrations of renin into the renal
circulation, and small quantities of angiotensin II could be formed
some way downstream. This might, for example, have a mild tonic
effect on superficial efferent arterioles, and help maintain filtration rate in these superficial nephrons.

The normal intrarenal distribution of renin is known to be
altered, for example, by sodium restriction or the application of
a renal artery clamp. In these circumstances, there is a general
increase in glomerular renin, affecting both superficial and deep
glomeruli, and considerable quantities are now found in association with the latter (Brown et al., 1966a, 1966b); Gavras et al.,
1970). A similar redistribution may well occur in other situations
such as haemorrhage, hypotension and cardiac failure. (After
glycerol injection, as we have seen (Figure 3) there is a general
reduction of glomerular renin. We suggest that this is a tempor-
ary response indicating discharge of renin into the circulation;
in the more chronic situation hypertrophy of the juxtaglomerular
cells, with increased formation, storage and release of renin,
could occur). Two consequences might follow:- more renin would
be formed and released throughout the renal circulation, and,

because of the more sluggish renal blood flow, effective concentrations of angiotensin II would be achieved more proximally, nearer
the renin storage site in the afferent glomerular arterioles. In
the superficial zones this could lead to narrowing or closure progressively of the glomerular capillaries or even eventually of the
afferent arterioles themselves, thus restricting the limited renal
blood supply progressively to the deeper glomeruli. In view of the
misunderstandings frequently associated with the work of Trueta et
al. (1947), it is emphasized that this does not imply any "shunting"
of blood from superficial to deep cortex. Indeed, juxtamedullary
blood flow could well be lower under these circumstances than in
normal conditions. The effect would, however, be initially to
improve deep nephron function in two ways. Increased tone and
consequent narrowing of the vasa recta would, by slowing the rate
of blood flow, initially improve the efficiency of the counter
current exchange systems, and so help maintain urea clearance (see
Brown et al., 1970b); and increased tone on efferent arterioles of
the deep glomeruli would increase their individual filtration rate.
This is close to the situation of moderately severe cardiac failure, in which there is a restriction of blood supply to superficial nephrons (see Barger, 1966), together with a well-maintained
filtration rate despite reduction in overall blood flow.

As renal blood flow became even more severely impaired, more
proximal vasoconstriction would affect the deep nephrons, whose
capillaries and even afferent arterioles, might close, and blood
urea would then rise steeply. A positive correlation between
blood urea and renin concentration would be expected in these
circumstances, and is particularly well seen in congestive cardiac
failure (Brown et al., 1970b; Figure 10).

With more severe impairment of renal function structural
damage in the form of necrosis affecting proximal, distal and
collecting tubules would appear, and evidence of glomerular damage might also be found (Clarkson et al., 1970). These structural
changes are known to be more severe in the renin-richest superficial areas of the cortex, and to spare the medulla and the
renin-free subcapsular zone.

SUMMARY AND CONCLUSIONS

The thoughts expressed in the last paragraph must be
regarded on present evidence as highly speculative. They are
offered as indicating one possible way in which acute circulatory
renal failure might develop as the pathological extreme of an
initially beneficial response to an impaired renal blood flow.

If renin and angiotensin are concerned in the pathogenesis
of acute renal failure, certain therapeutic implications follow.

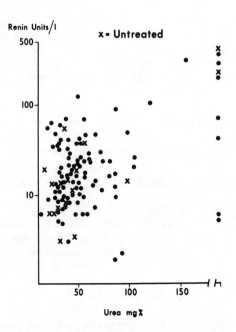

Figure 10. Relationship between peripheral venous plasma renin
            concentration and concurrent blood urea level in
            congestive cardiac failure. Log. ordinate scale.
            Urea values greater than 190 mg per cent plotted to
            right of break in abscissa. Crosses indicate untreat-
            ed cases; dots treated cases. r = +0.97 for untreated;
            +0.57 for whole group; p < 0.001 for both.

The effects of saline-loading in protecting against renal failure
have already been discussed. Conversely, measures likely to
increase circulating renin and angiotensin levels (such as surgery,
sodium deprivation or diuretic administration), should, on present
evidence, be avoided or undertaken with caution, in cases of
established or impending acute renal failure.

     In summary, peripheral levels of renin, renin activity and
angiotensin are consistently elevated in clinical acute renal failure, subsiding as the renal function improves.

     In glycerol-induced renal failure in the rabbit, plasma renin
concentration is also increased, the peak level of renin slightly
preceding the peak blood urea value.

     By contrast, in cephaloridine-induced renal failure in the
rabbit, peripheral arterial plasma renin concentration is not significantly raised. These findings do not exclude a contributory

role of renin and angiotensin in cephaloridine-induced renal
failure, however, since experiments in which tubular necrosis was
induced by renal artery clamping show that very marked increases
in renal venous plasma renin concentration can occur in the absence
of a detectable change in arterial plasma renin when the renal
blood flow is greatly reduced.

The intravenous infusion of large doses of angiotensin II
consistently produces acute renal failure and tubular necrosis in
the rabbit. The tubular lesions resemble those induced by subcutaneous glycerol or by renal artery clamping, being more widespread
than the cephaloridine-induced lesions, which are localised to
proximal tubules.

Angiotensin infusion also produces focal myocardial infarction
in the rabbit. That comparable myocardial lesions may occur in
some clinical situations in man is also considered possible.

REFERENCES

Akinkugbe, O.O., Brown, W.C.B., Cranston, W.I. (1966). Clin. Sci.,
    30, 409.
Bailie, M.D., Rector, F.C., Seldin, D.W. (1971). J. Clin. Invest.,
    50, 119.
Barger, A.C. (1966). Ann. New York Acad. Sci., 139, 276.
Barger, A.C., Herd, J.A. (1971). New Engl. Med. J., 284, 482.
Bock, K.D., Brown, J.J., Lever, A.F., Robertson, J.I.S. (1968)
    In Renal Hypertension. Eds. I.H. Page & J.W. McCubbin, p. 184.
    Year Book Publishers, Chicago.
Brown, J.J., Chapuis, G., Robertson, J.I.S. (1964a). Clin. Sci.,
    26, 165.
Brown, J.J., Davies, D.L., Lever, A.F., Robertson, J.I.S. (1964b).
    J. Physiol., 170, 408.
Brown, J.J., Davies, D.L., Lever, A.F., Parker, R.A., Robertson,
    J.I.S. (1965). J. Physiol., 176, 418.
Brown, J.J., Davies, D.L., Lever, A.F., Robertson, J.I.S. (1966a).
    Postgrad. Med. J., 42, 153.
Brown, J.J., Davies, D.L., Lever, A.F., Parker, R.A., Robertson,
    J.I.S. (1966b). Clin. Sci., 30, 223.
Brown, J.J., Davies, D.L., Lever, A.F., Robertson, J.I.S.,
    Bianchi, G., Imbs, J.L., Johnston, V.W., Lawrence, M., Fraser,
    R., James, V.H.T. (1967). Proc. 3rd Int. Congr. Nephrol.,
    Vol. 1, p. 226. Edited by Handler, J.S.,Karger, Basel and
    New York.
Brown, J.J., Fraser, R., Lever, A.F., Robertson, J.I.S. (1968).
    In Recent Advances in Endocrinology, 8th edition, edited by
    V.H.T. James, p. 271. Churchill, London.

Brown, J.J., Gleadle, R.I., Lawson, D.H., Lever, A.F., Linton, A.L.,
    MacAdam, R., Prentice, E., Robertson, J.I.S., Tree, M. (1970a).
    Brit. Med. J., 1, 253.
Brown, J.J., Davies, D.L., Lever, A.F., Johnson, V.W., Robertson,
    J.I.S. (1970b). Amer. Ht. J., 80, 329.
Brown, J.J., Düsterdieck, G., Fraser, R., Lever, A.F., Robertson,
    J.I.S., Tree, M., Weir, R.J. (1971a). Brit. Med. Bull., 27,
    128.
Brown, W.C.B., Brown, J.J., Gavras, H., Jackson, A., MacAdam, R.,
    Robertson, J.I.S. (1971b). Circ. Res. (in press).
Brun, C., Munck, O. (1957). Lancet, 1, 603.
Byrom, F.B. (1964). Brit. J. Exp. Path., 45, 7.
Carrière, S., Biron, P. (1970). Am. J. Physiol., 219, 1642.
Clarkson, A.R., MacDonald, M.K., Fuster, V., Cash, J.D., Robson,
    J.M. (1970). Quart. J. Med., 39, 585.
Cook, W.F. (1971). In Kidney Hormones. Ed. J.W. Fisher. p. 117.
    Academic Press, London and New York.
Daniel, P.M., Prichard, M.M.L., Ward-McQuaid, J.N. (1954). J.
    Physiol., 124, 106.
Davis, J.O. (1961). Rec. Progr. Horm. Res., 17, 293.
Davis, J.O. (1971). In Kidney Hormones, edited by J.W. Fisher.
    p. 173. Academic Press, London and New York.
De Bono, E., Lee, G., Mottram, F., Pickering, G.W., Brown, J.J.,
    Keen, H., Peart, W.S., Sanderson, P.H. (1963). Clin. Sci.,
    25, 123.
De Wardener, H.E. (1963). The Kidney. 2nd edition, p. 127.
    Churchill, London.
Düsterdieck, G., McElwee, G. (1971). Europ. J. Clin. Invest.,
    (in press).
Finckh, E.S., Jeremy, D., Whyte, H.M. (1962). Quart. J. Med., 31,
    429.
Fitzsimons, J.T., Simons, B.J. (1969). J. Physiol., 203, 45.
Gavras, H., Brown, J.J., Lever, A.F., Robertson, J.I.S. (1970).
    Clin. Sci., 38, 409.
Gavras, H., Brown, J.J., Lever, A.F., MacAdam, R., Robertson,
    J.I.S. (1971a). Lancet, 2, 19.
Gavras, H., Brown, J.J., Lawson, D.H., Lever, A.F., MacAdam, R.F.,
    Robertson, J.I.S. (1971b). (Unpublished).
Genest, J., Nowaczynski, W., Koiw, E., Sandor, P., Biron, P.
    (1960). In Essential Hypertension, edited by K.D. Bock and
    P.T. Cottier, p. 126. Springer-Verlag, Berlin.
Gocke, D.J., Gerten, J., Sherwood, L.M., Laragh, J.H. (1969).
    Circ. Res., 24-25, Suppl. I, 131.
Goormaghtigh, N. (1942). Bull. Acad. Roy. Med. Belg., 7, 194.
Goormaghtigh, N. (1945). Proc. Soc. Exp. Biol. Med., 59, 303.
Goormaghtigh, N. (1947). Am. J. Path., 23, 513.
Gross, F. (1958). Klin. Wschr., 36, 693.
Gross, F. (1960). In Essential Hypertension. Edited by K.D. Bock
    and P.T. Cottier, p. 92. Springer-Verlag, Berlin.

Gross, F., Schaechtelin, G., Brunner, H., Peters, G. (1964).
    Canad. Med. Ass. J., 90, 258.
Helmer, O.M., Judson, W.E. (1967). Am. J. Obs. Gyn., 99, 9.
Henry, L.N., Lane, C.E., Kashgarian, M. (1968). Lab. Invest., 19,
    309.
Hosie, K.F., Brown, J.J., Harper, A.M., McGregor, J., Robertson,
    J.I.S. (1970). Clin. Sci., 38, 157.
Kokot, F., Kuska, J. (1969). Nephron., 6, 115.
Ladefoged, J., Munck, O. (1971). In Kidney Hormones, edited by
    J.W. Fisher. p. 31. Academic Press, London and New York.
Laragh, J.H., Angers, M., Kelly, W.G., Lieberman, S. (1960). J.
    Amer. Med. Ass., 174, 234.
Lever, A.F., Peart, W.S. (1962). J. Physiol., 160, 548.
Massani, Z.M., Finkielman, S., Worcel, M., Agrest, A., Paladini,
    A.C. (1966). Clin. Sci., 30, 473.
Mulrow, P.J., Ganong, W.F. (1961). Yale J. Biol. Med., 33, 386.
Ng, K.F., Vane, J.R. (1968). Nature, 218, 144.
Ochoa, E., Finkielman, S., Agrest, A. (1970). Clin. Sci., 38, 225.
Oken, D.E., Arce, M.L., Wilson, D.R. (1966). J. Clin. Invest., 45,
    724.
Oliver, J., MacDowell, M.C., Tracey, A. (1951). J. Clin. Invest.,
    30, 1307.
Oparil, S., Sanders, C.A., Haber, E. (1970). Circ. Res., 26, 591.
Pickering, G.W., Prinzmetal, M. (1938). Clin. Sci., 3, 211.
Pickering, G.W., Prinzmetal, M. (1940). J. Physiol. 98, 314.
Powers, S.R., Boba, A., Stein, A. (1957). Surgery, 42, 156.
Robertson, J.I.S., Weir, R.J., Düsterdieck, G.O., Fraser, R., Tree,
    M. (1971). Scott. Med. J., 16, 183.
Roguska, J., Del Greco, F., Simon, N.M. (1971). Nephron., 8, 289.
Schröder, E., Herms, W., Wetzels, E., Dume, T., Grabensee, B.
    (1969). Deuts. Med. Wchsr., 44, 2262.
Schroeder, E.T., Eich, R.H., Smulyan, H., Gould, A.B., Gabuzda,
    G.J. (1970). Am. J. Med., 49, 186.
Sevitt, S. (1959). Lancet, 2, 135.
Sundsfjord, J.A. (1969). Lancet, 2, 807.
Teschan, P.E., Lawson, N.L. (1966). Nephron., 3, 1.
Thurau, K., Dahlheim, H., Granger, P. (1970). Proc. 4th Int. Congr.
    Nephrol., Stockholm, Vol. 2, p. 24. Edited by Alwall, N.,
    Berglund, F. and Josephson, B.,Karger, Basel and New York.
Tigerstedt, R., Bergman, P.G. (1898). Skand. Arch. Physiol., 8, 223.
Trueta, J., Barclay, A.E., Daniel, P.M., Franklin, K.J., Prichard,
    M.M.L. (1947). Studies of the renal circulation. Blackwell,
    Oxford.
Tu, W.H. (1965). Circulation, 31, 686.
Ueda, H., Tagawa, H., Ishii, M., Kaneko, Y. (1967) Jap. Heart J.,
    8, 156.
Wilson, D.R., Thiel, G., Arce, M.L., Oken, D.E. (1967). Nephron.,
    4, 337.

INDEX

Adrenal denervation, 17
Adrenalectomy, 25,27,68-70,78,123-124
Aldosterone
  biosynthesis, 172
  control of, 167-184
    by angiotensin metabolites, 184
    by central nervous system, 175,178-181
    by potassium, 174-175,182
    by renin, 167-168
    during sodium deficiency, 169-184
  excretion, 210-213,220-221
  half-life, 232-235,248
  metabolic clearance rate, 232-235,238,248
  plasma concentration, 237-238
  secretion, 219,222,230-231,237-238,245-260
  volume of distribution, 232-235
Aldosteronism, primary, 210,220,223-224
Alpha adrenergic receptors (see phentolamine;phenoxybenzamine)
Alpha-methyldopa, 93-100
Angiotensin, administration of, 109-115,169-175,257,259,272-274
Angiotensinase, 134,136,140
Angiotensinogen (see renin substrate)
Aortic constriction, 118,120,122-123
Area postrema, 109-115

Baroreceptors, 117-128
Beta adrenergic receptors (see propranolol)
Blood pressure, 55-56,60,66-77,84-85,87-89,104-105,107-115,122,
    163-165,198-200,204,249-250,252,257
Brain, 17-18,103-108,109-115

Cardiac output, 55-56,60-61
Congestive heart failure, 227-241,282-283

Converting enzyme
   hindlimb, 154-155
   juxtaglomerular apparatus, 134,136,140
   kidney, 154-156
   liver, 154-155
   lung, 154-156
   lymph, 137,140
   plasma, 151-154
Cyclic nucleotides, 18,33-45

Disappearance rate, 202,205
Diurnal rhythmicity, 189-191

Epinephrine, 18,127-128
Exercise, 230-235
Extracellular fluid volume, 218,224

Furosemide, 24-26

Hematocrit, 57,59,61
Hemodialysis, 193-207
Hemorrhage, 66-68,77-78,117-119,121-127
Hypercalciurea, 245-262
Hypertension
   accelerated, 209-215
   essential, 84,199
   low renin, 217-225
   malignant, 209-215
   post-salt, 159
      and interstitial cells of renal medulla, 160-165
   "refractory", 193-207
   renovascular, 84,209-215,277
Hypoglycemia, 17

Interstitial cells (see renal medulla)
Intrarenal role of renin, 131-142,263-284
Isoproterenol, 33,53-62

Juxtaglomerular apparatus
   anatomy, 1-13
   angiotensinase activity, 134,136,140
   converting enzyme, 134,136,140,278-279
   electron microscopy, 1-13,137-138,141
   hyperplasia, 254,259
   innervation, 10-13
   protogranules, 2-4
   renin content, 134-135,137-141,269

Kidney, beta receptors in, 18-22

Kidney, non-filtering, 117-128
Kidney slices, renin release by, 145-149

Liver function, 232,236
Lymph (see renal lymph)

Macula densa, 117-128,137-141
  relationship to efferent and afferent arterioles, 7-10
Medulla oblongata, 17-18,103-108,109-115
Methylnorepinephrine, 98,100
Myocardial infarction, 274-276

Norepinephrine, 18,97-98,100,127-128,224,237,239

Oral contraceptives, 211,220
Osmolality, and renin release in vitro, 148-149

Papaverine, 124-128
Pentobarbital anesthesia, 23-24
Phenoxybenzamine, 17-21,28,33,53,88-89
Phentolamine, 66-80,88
Posture, 83-90,93,95,195,197-199,203-204,209-213
Potassium
  plasma levels, 21,41-44,53,57,59,60,212-215,219,249-260
  urinary excretion, 42,57,58,212-215,222-223,245-250,252-253,256
Propranolol, 17-30,33,53,67-80,84-90
Prostaglandin, 162-166,181

Renal artery constriction, 72-77,79,89,97-99,271-272
Renal disease, end stage, 193-207
Renal failure, acute, 264-284
Renal function, 42-43,45,57-58,61,72-77,98-99,123,237,239
Renal lymph, 137,140
Renal medulla, interstitial cells of, 159-166
  antihypertensive effect of, 162-165
  lipid granules in, 160-162
  prostaglandin in, 162-166
Renal nerves
  denervation, 17-18,25,27,53,56,97,121-127,175,177
  direct effect on renin release, 126-127
  innervation of juxtaglomerular apparatus, 10-13
  stimulation, 18-20,94,96-97,100,104-105,107-108,126-127
Renal papilla (see renal medulla)
Renal renin, 269
Renin accelerator, 202
Renin inhibitor, 197,201,205
Renin substrate
  lymph, 137
  plasma, 117-120,122-123,197-198,200,205,218

Sodium
  concentration in distal tubule, 137-140
  deficiency, 27-29,70-72,78-79,85-88,134-135,140,146,148,189-191,
     199,210,218-224,249-250,252-253,256-260
    paradoxical response, 210-215
  effect on in vitro renin release, 146-147,149
  exchangeable, 218
  loading, 134-135,140,199,203,210,218-224,249-250,252-253,256-260
    paradoxical response, 210-215
  plasma levels, 57,59
  urinary excretion, 57-58,220-223
Sympathetic nervous system, 17-30,33-45,49-62,65-80,83-90,93-100,
    103-108,121-128

Theophylline, 18,33,41-42,44-45,50-53,57,59-60

Vertebral artery embolism, 103-108